MEAL PREP

This Book Contains 2 Manuscripts :

1) <u>Vegetarian Meal Prep</u>

2) <u>Vegan Meal Prep</u>

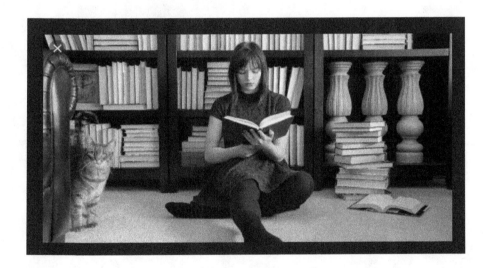

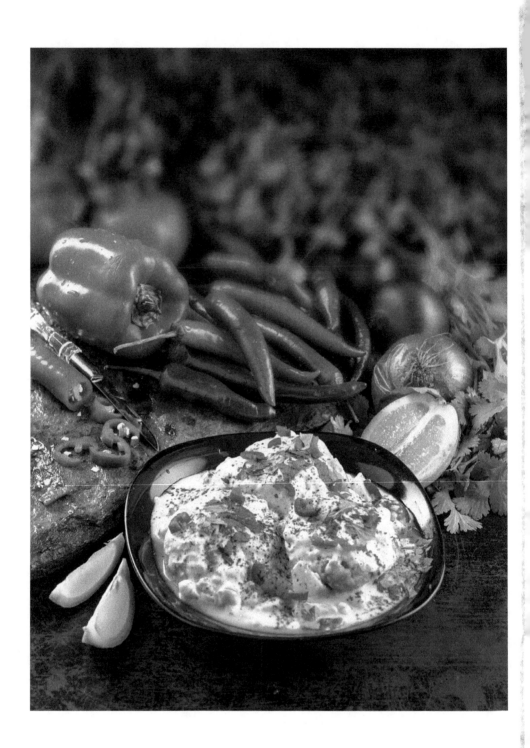

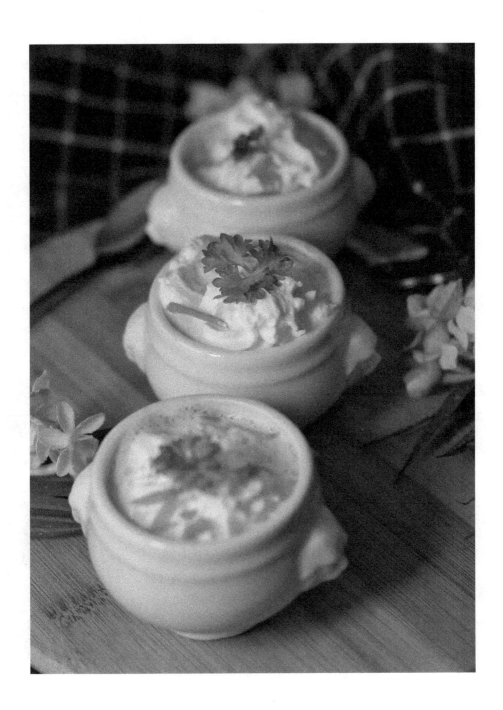

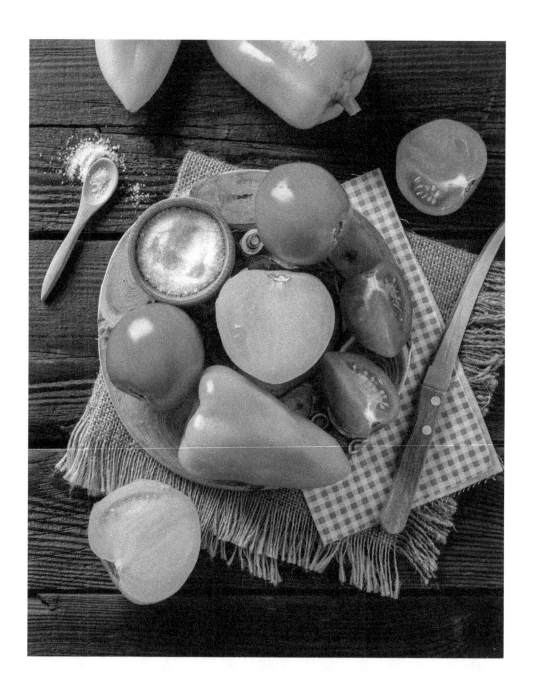

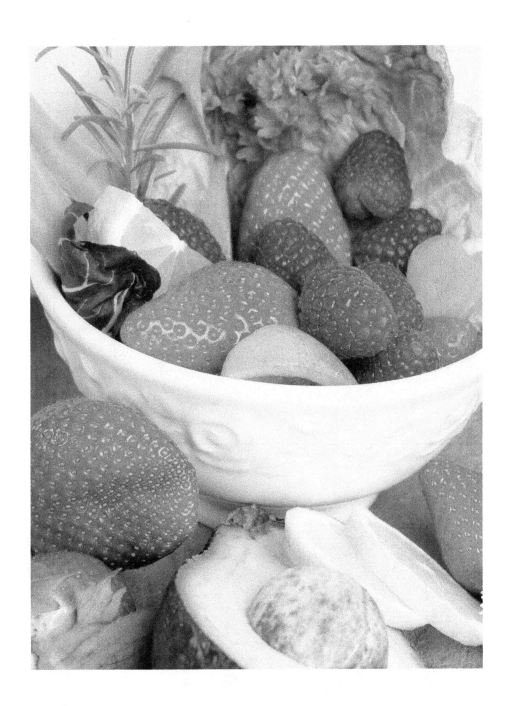

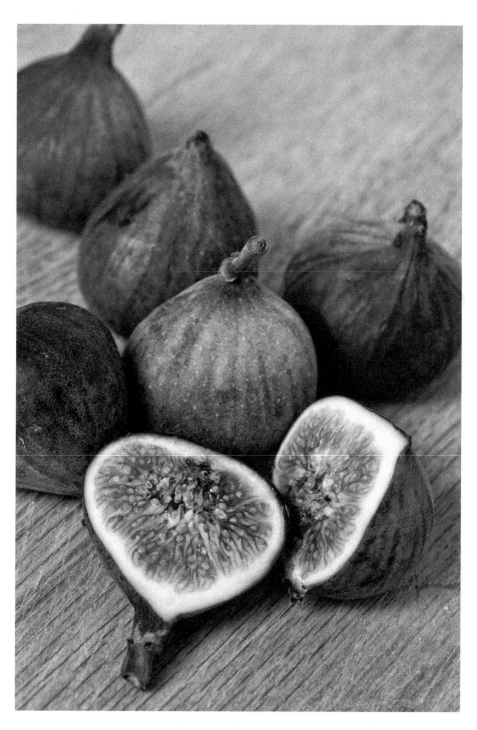

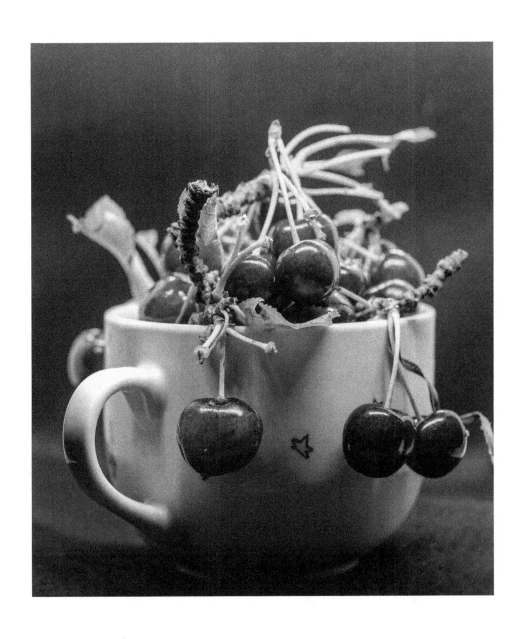

**Read this book today and find out
how to meal prep fast for a healthy lifestyle !**

Vegetarian Meal Prep

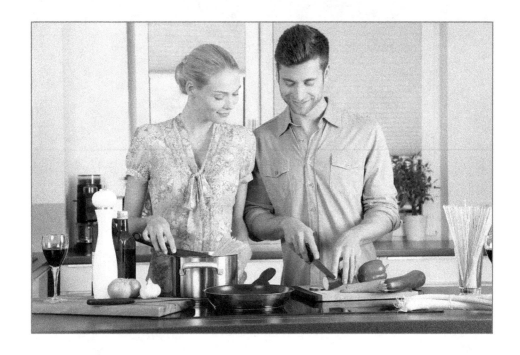

A Complete Vegetarian Meal Prep Book, For Weight Loss And Increase Energy. Top Foods For Breakfast, Lunch, And Dinner. Easy To Be Made And Great Taste.

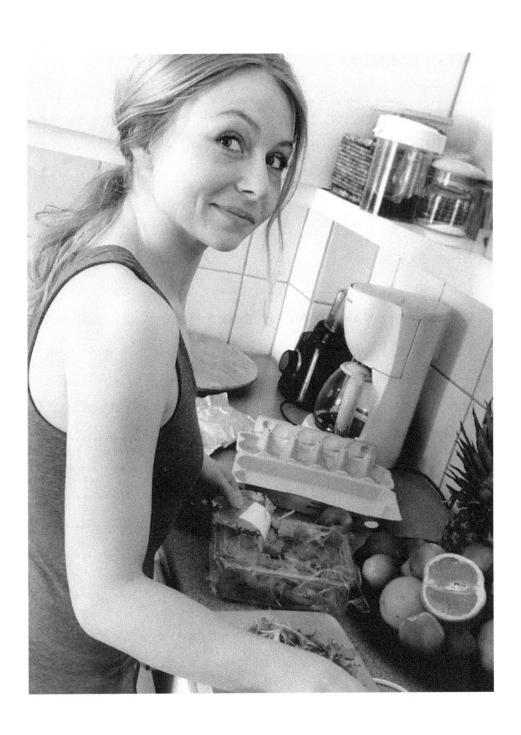

TABLE OF CONTENTS

Description

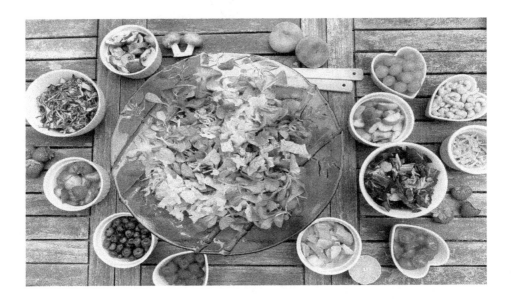

If you want to create a healthy, sustainable vegetarian lifestyle and not break the bank or lose your free time while doing it, then keep reading!

- Do you want to save time and money at the grocery store each week without compromising quality and taste of your food?

- Are you tired of cooking and want to free yourself from being chained to the stove every day while still enjoying tasty meals that are great for you?

- Do you wish you had a guidebook to help you learn how to do this without spending hours looking for recipes?

- Our fresh, hot, delectable meals something you want to have for every occasion instead of having to depend on the drive-through because you are tired after a long day?

This book will teach you everything you need to know to get started and prepare scrumptious vegetarian meals that are good for you without having to spend hours to do them! Learn about what meal prep is, how it will help you save time and money, and how to get started doing it today. If you want to get healthy, lose weight, and feel great while keeping up with a vegetarian lifestyle, this book is for you!

Inside this book you will find

- Lists of all the equipment you will need to get started preparing meals and a bonus list of items to invest in that will make your life easier.

- Tricks on how to save yourself time in the kitchen so you can have more free time to do the things you love.

- A guide to make grocery shopping simple, easy, and fast instead of the boring chore it once was.

- Tips for customizing your meal prep to work best for you, your lifestyle, and the type of foods you like to eat.

- Recommendations on how to create unique flavor combinations that make your taste buds water and let eat at home instead of eating out.

- Recipes for breakfast, lunch, dinner, and snacks that are ready to go, easy to make, and taste great.

Never tried a vegetarian diet? No problem! This book provides plenty of great vegetarian recipes for every meal and snacks. If you want to lose weight and live a healthier lifestyle, this book is where you need to start!

Even if your week is already swamped and you feel like you have no more time to devote to a new routine, you can quickly and easily learn how to turn your daily cooking grind into a once per week event that will give you the time to focus on the things you care about. With this simple, ready to use the guide you can transform your food from being boring and exhausting to prepare into the delight of your day and something you were looking for!

Introduction

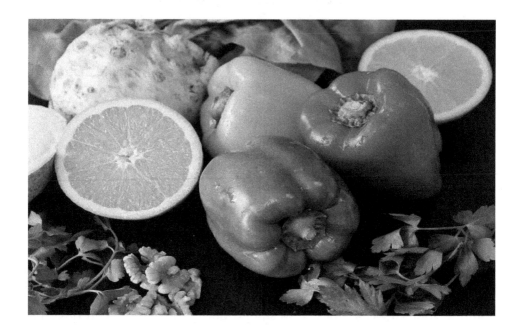

Congratulations on buying : **"Vegetarian Meal Prepping"**

The Exclusive Guide for Ready-to-Go Meals for a Healthy Plant-Based Whole Foods Diet with a 30-Day Time- and Money-Saving Easy Meal Plan.

Thank you for doing so and for your decision to pursue a sustainable and healthy vegetarian lifestyle. Your body, wallet, and the weekly schedule will thank you for it!

The chapters included in this book will teach you all about how to make meal prep work for you to reduce the amount of time you spend in the kitchen each week while still eating good vegetarian food that tastes great.

This book starts by discussing the basics of meal prep, including descriptions of what meal prep is, different options for how to prepare meals to best suit your lifestyle and the type of foods you like to eat, and the equipment you will need to get started with prepping meals.

As a bonus, you will also receive a list of life-changing items for the kitchen that will make preparing meals an absolute breeze.

After that, you will learn about how to plan your menu to include healthy vegetarian meals all week long, tips for making grocery shopping a cinch and how to save money while at the store, and a list of suggestions that will save you time in the shopping and prepping process.

Finally, you will receive a plethora of tasty recipes for every meal and snacks that can easily be made once a week (or sometimes less!) that will provide you with hot, delicious food whenever you want it.

There are plenty of books on this subject on the market, so thanks again for choosing this one! Every effort was made to ensure it is as full of as much useful information as possible! Please enjoy!

Chapter One
Meal Prep Basics

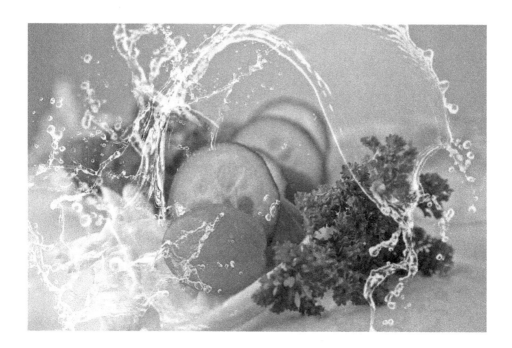

Everything you need to know about getting started and what you'll need to start saving time and money on healthy meals that taste great

Why to prepare meals?

Do you come from work and dread cooking after an exhausting day? Do you find yourself reaching for whatever is quick and easy rather than healthy food options? Are you constantly running out of time or feeling rushed? Have you tried eating a healthy vegetarian diet but had trouble sticking with it?

If the answer is yes, then meal prep is perfect for you! By prepping meals in advance, you can save yourself time and money, eat better, and take the stress out of the question, "What's for dinner?" Meal prep is the key to making healthy, homecooked, and tasty meals every day! Prepping meals for the week all at once saves you time in the kitchen every day.

Instead of spending 30 minutes to an hour cooking daily, you can get everything done at once and relax in the evenings! Not only that, but you will save yourself hundreds of dollars on your grocery bills by only buying what you will use in your meals throughout the week.

By taking charge of your menu, you make it easier on yourself to stick with healthy vegetarian options instead of turning to what's quick and easy (which means it's probably not good for you!). By freeing yourself of the constant need to make decisions about meals, you can focus more time and energy on more important things!

How do I do it?

Meal prep can look scary or intimidating when you're first getting started, but it's very simple! There are several different methods you can use:

- Preparing ingredients: This is the most basic method, where you would chop, slice, and dice all your veggies, proteins, and garnishes.

You can also make marinades, sauces, or spice mixes to make your food taste great. Then everything you need is ready to go for a fresh, hot meal every day.

- Single-serve meals: Cook a big batch of something tasty and divvy it up into single-serving containers. This also works great for chopping veggies for salads or portioning out healthy snacks and desserts.

- Full meals in advance: Enjoy variety? With this method, you make your meals all at once and store them in containers for each day. Then you aren't limited to a single option.

- Freezer-ready: If you enjoy foods that are easy to make in large batches, this is the way to go! It is perfect for soups, stews, rice, and curries, or for freezing fruits that are in season for smoothies or just to munch when you're craving something sweet.

What do I need?

Meal prep supplies come in two varieties: must-haves and time-saving extras. You probably have almost all of the must-haves in your kitchen already, so getting started should be a breeze. It's always a good idea to invest in high-quality equipment, especially for something you do often. While cheaper options can get you started and get you by for a little while, they tend to break or dull a lot sooner than the equipment you spend a little more money on.

Using high-quality equipment will also reduce the amount of time you need to spend doing things like cutting veggies or grating cheeses. Must-haves:

- **Containers:** Containers are the cornerstone of meal prep. Since you're portioning out food for an entire week, you need to make sure you have enough containers for every meal. Choosing containers that can stack or are similar in size or shape will help you fit everything into your fridge or freezer. There are several different options as far as containers go:

  - **Glass jars:** These babies are amazingly versatile! They are fantastic for layered salads for lunches, storing chopped ingredients with an airtight seal so they don't brown or go bad, or for freezing (just make sure you leave enough room at the top for any liquids to expand!)

  - **Silicone:** Silicone containers are microwavable, so you can heat an entire meal in a jiffy. These are also often collapsible, which makes packing up after lunch or storing them a breeze!

  - **Divided BPA-free containers:** This is your go-to for dinners! Using divided containers makes it easy to ensure you're eating a balanced diet and getting enough protein, vegetables, and whole grains at every meal.

o **Reusable bags:** Also great for anything that needs an airtight seal or to go in the freezer. But these bags also have the benefit of taking up less space, so you can store more.

- **Knives:** Never overlook the importance of having good kitchen knives! A sharp, high-quality knife will cut down the amount of time and effort you need to put into cutting, chopping, and dicing. Having special knives for specific purposes will make this even easier.

    o **Chef's knife:** This is your all-in-one knife that can do just about any job in the kitchen. If you can only invest in one knife, make it this one! It can slice, chop, and make fine cuts and is great for any fruit, veggie, or protein you come across.

    o **Paring knife:** Smaller than a chef's knife, a paring knife is perfect for removing the peels or rinds from veggies and fruits. You can also use it to create garnishes to go with your meals.

    o **Kitchen shears:** These are not your ordinary scissors! Kitchen shears are used for snipping fresh herbs, dicing veggies fast, or even cutting pizza!

- **Cutting boards:** Cutting boards are an often overlooked yet vital component to every kitchen. When you are preparing ingredients for an entire week's worth of meals at once, they become even more important. They will save your kitchen counters, your knives, and your food from damage. It's best to have at least 3 in different sizes, preferably small, medium, and large so that you can fit anything from a carrot to an entire watermelon on one!

- **Mixing bowls:** Along with blending ingredients, mixing bowls are essential for marinating veggies before they go in the oven. You will want a variety of sizes so you can have multiple bowls going at once and accommodate foods of any size and shape. Glass bowls are best, but metal bowls are also good choices.

- **Measuring cups and spoons:** You can't make a recipe if you don't know how much of something to add! The more sizes you have of these, the easier your life will be. You can also find collapsible silicone versions to save space in your drawers.

- **Baking sheets:** Using the oven is one of the best ways to cook veggies that taste great. Once you pop the tray in the oven and set your timer, you can move onto other things without having to constantly stir. A large baking tray will fit enough veggies at once for an entire week's worth of dinners, or you can use two smaller trays side-by-side to cook multiple veggies at the same time.

- **Cooling rack:** It's important to let your food cool before packing it up and storing it in the fridge or freezer. The fastest way to do this is to use a cooling rack. It's also the best way to prevent excess moisture from building up on your food.

- **Grater:** Grating your fresh cheese instead of buying packaged is the first thing that comes to mind, but a grater is so much more versatile than just this. You can use it for veggies to go on salads or adding zested lemons or another citrus to kick the flavor of your meals up to a notch. Once you use your grater to utilize fresh spices like cinnamon and taste the difference yourself, you'll never go back to jars again.

Time-saving extras:

- **Rice cooker:** This one piece of equipment will save you hours! Rice is a wonderful and filling staple to add to any meal, but it can take so long to cook. Using a rice cooker instead of having to constantly stir and check to make sure it is not burned or hard in the middle will take the headache out of cooking rice once and for all.

- **Crockpot:** A crockpot is a fantastic way to cook a large batch of stew or curry. You can also use this piece of equipment to make sure you have a fresh, hot meal ready to go when you get home at the end of the day. By adding prepared ingredients and leaving on low temperature for several hours,

22

you can start dinner first thing in the morning before you leave and not have to wait for it once you get home. Crockpots are not just for dinners, either! You can make some tasty treats, like cakes, puddings, or cobblers in a crockpot.

- **Food processor:** A food processor will cut the time you spend chopping down to nothing. Most food processors have several different blades, which can provide a variety of results. You can do anything from creating veggie noodles to dicing onions (without the tears!) to pureeing salsa.

- **Blender:** Not just for smoothies or milkshakes. Blenders are great for creating homemade marinades or sauces. You can even make your peanut or almond butter in one! Bullet-style blenders are an especially good choice for meal prep. They come with large and small blender jars, as well as lids and shaker tops!

- **Food scale:** A scale is a more precise way to measure ingredients than measuring cups or spoons. It is also handy for separating proper portion sizes or if you happen to find a European recipe you want to try.

- **Mandolin:** No, not the instrument! A mandolin is a quick, easy way to slice fruits and veggies. Like a food processor, most come with a variety of different blades to produce different types of cuts. A good mandolin will also have a high adjustment knob so you can create slices as thick or as thin as you want them.

- **Garlic press:** Just about any food tastes better when you add a bit of fresh garlic but mincing it can be tedious and time-consuming. A garlic press takes a task that seems to take forever and make it happen in an instant.

- **Hand blender:** Also known as a stick mixer, this bad boy can mix anything from smoothies to soups. It's great for use with smaller pots and bowls since it is more compact than your traditional hand mixer. You can also quickly and easily blend spices.

- **Vegetable peeler:** Instead of painstakingly using a knife to peel potatoes, just use a vegetable peeler instead. A few quick motions will remove any peel without having to press very hard.

- **Food dehydrator:** Dehydrated fruits and veggies make great healthy snacks, but they can take a long time to make in the oven since they require low temperatures and take up precious oven space you need for roasting veggies. A food dehydrator accomplishes this easily, and you can stack several different fruits, veggies, or both in as many or as few trays as you want.

Vacuum sealer: This gadget is helps creat an airtight seal around any food, even ones that are too large or oddly shaped to fit in a regular sealable bag. Vacuum seals guarantee freshness and will help packages of prepared foods fit more easily in the freezer.

- **Hot water kettle:** Rather than having to wait around for water to boil on the stove, a water kettle makes the process go so much faster. This is great for making foods like hardboiled eggs or for pouring into a larger pot to cook noodles fast.

- **Plastic tubs:** These go in your fridge and pantry for easy storage and sorting. You can have one for snacks, one for seasonings, another for pasta... Your imagination is the limit!

- **Fatigue reduction kitchen mat:** Prepping meals can mean standing in one spot for a while. A fatigue reduction mat makes this easier on your body. Your feet, knees, and back will thank you for this addition to your kitchen.

Chapter Two
Making Meal Prep a Habit

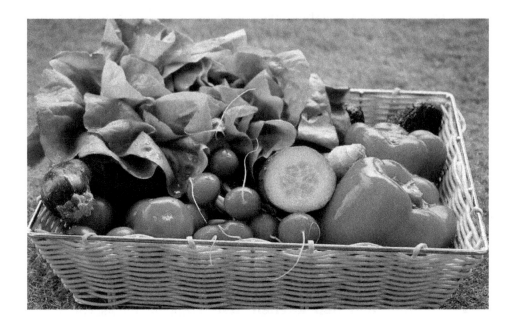

Tips and tricks for creating a sustainable, healthy vegetarian lifestyle

Planning your menu

Menu planning is probably the single most important part of prepping healthy, great-tasting meals. Without a menu, it's hard to know what ingredients to buy and you are more likely to be tempted by options that are not very good for you.

Planning a menu ahead of time helps you make sure you are getting enough of all the macronutrients you need and will save you money once you're at the store.

Ensuring you are getting your macronutrients in the right proportions is especially important for vegetarians since it can sometimes be challenging to make sure you are eating enough protein and not eating too many carbohydrates.

How to start planning your menu:

- Begin with plans for dinner options. This is where the majority of people like to have the most variety in their meals, so it can be the most difficult one to plan for. Dinners also usually require the most ingredients, so having a plan for this can give you an idea of things you can buy in bulk and use for breakfast or lunch to save money.

- Take care of lunch ideas after planning for dinners. If you enjoy cooking food in bulk to reduce the amount of cooking you have to do, many of your dinner options can double for lunch, but in smaller portion sizes. You could also use specific elements of your dinner ingredients, such as the veggies, to make some spectacular salads that won't get boring.

- Think about breakfast next. Breakfast is the most important meal of the day, so you should never skip it! Treat it as the vital start to the day that it is. Breakfasts can be sweet or savory, so you have no end of tasty options.

- Finally, plan for snacks and desserts. This is a step that many people forget to do, but it can make or break a healthy diet.

Everyone gets cravings or can become hungry outside of mealtime, so having prepared, healthy snacks is the secret to success for sustaining good eating habits.

When planning out your menu, make sure to include exactly the number of meals you will need. If you plan to have a night of eating out, you need to make sure to consider that when preparing your menu so that you don't buy too much food when you go shopping. Snacks can be the hardest to plan for the right amount with, so this may take some experimentation before you know what works best for you. Until then, it's a good idea to keep packets of slices fruits or veggies handy since they are good to eat anytime.

There is more than one way to plan your menu, so this is where you can add some of your styles into meal prep.

- **Dinner options**
  - Plan a different meal every night. If possible, ensure this something you can make extra to use for lunches as well.
  - Choose one meal to make in a large batch, like a curry, and eat this for 3-4 nights in a week. Alternate this with nights of different meals to keep variety in your diet.
  - Pick two recipes that can make large batches and alternate them. This option is the most budget-friendly, but you will want to make sure you choose recipes you enjoy so you don't get bored with them by the end of the week.
- **Lunch options**
  - Lunches should be quick, easy, and simple, so the best option here is to choose one recipe for the entire week. You can change things up by having something a little different on the weekends as a treat.
  - If you make different meals every night for dinner, you can plan to cook a little bit more than absolutely needed and use the "leftovers" for lunch. This will ensure that your midday meal stays interesting.
  - Like with dinners, choose two options and alternate them during the week, even on the weekends.
- **Breakfast options**
  - Pick a theme for the week and make variations on that theme for every day. For example, have toast or oatmeal every day, but change the toppings you add to it for different flavor profiles.

- Choose one sweet and one savory recipe for the week and alternate throughout the week. This gives you the best of both breakfast worlds.
- Choose one recipe to eat during the week and another recipe for the weekends. This way you can plan something that's a bit of a treat for your relaxing weekend days.

- **Snacks**
  - Choose at least 3-4 snack recipes for a week. This is the area you are most likely to "cheat" on, so having a variety can help you stay on track.
  - The one exception to this rule is dessert. Plan to make one dessert or sweet snack that you will eat all week long, but make sure to portion properly!
  - Ensure that you have snacks on hand with different flavor profiles to combat any sort of craving you may have. These include savory, salty, sweet, and spicy. Spicy snacks will also help give your metabolism a boost, keeping your body in top calorie-burning shape.

Grocery shopping

Once you start prepping meals in advance, grocery shopping is no longer the headache it was before! It will take less time to complete and you won't come home with ingredients or foods you don't end up using that just clutter up your cabinets. As you are writing down your recipes for the week, start a grocery list based on the ingredients.

By writing your grocery list as you plan your menu, you will eliminate the need to go back through your recipes again and save yourself time in the process.

Decide on which grocery store you will shop at before you leave the house to go shopping. Then order your list based on how the store is arranged. This will reduce the amount of walking you do in the store and is another way to save yourself time, which is what meal prep is all about. This way you can also check sales brochures and look for coupons to save yourself even more money than you already are.

One trick to ensuring you have plenty of healthy ingredients for your meals is to focus on the ones around the edge of the store and ignore the shelves in the middle. The foods on the outside of the store tend to be the freshest and healthiest, while the foods in the center aisles are usually packed full of chemicals, preservatives, and other additives that are not very healthy or good for you.

Try to focus on fruits and vegetables that are ripe at the time you are shopping. These will be the freshest, taste the best, and will usually be the least expensive options for your meals. By planning your ingredients by season, you will also be able to rotate through different recipes regularly(but not so often that it gets overwhelming!) to keep variety in your meals and continue making prepared meals interesting. Shopping at a store that has a bulk foods section will save you a TON of money. This way you can get as much or as little of specific ingredients as you want to minimize waste or maximize your savings.

This is a great way to stock up on essentials like rice, flour, oats, and granola. You can also find a wide variety of nuts in bulk food sections, which are a wonderful source of protein for vegetarians and make fantastic snacks. You can eat them plain or toss them with your favorite seasonings to have a variety of flavors on hand during the week.

Don't go grocery shopping on the same day that you plan on prepping your meals if you can help it. Both tasks can take up at least an hour or two of your day, so trying to both on the same day can become tiring. Spreading them out will make you more likely to stick with the habit of preparing meals instead of becoming frustrated with how much time it takes to do.

Similarly, don't go grocery shopping when you're hungry. If you are already thinking about food, you are more likely to buy impulsively and add items that are not on your list. This will cost you extra money and your food choices when you are hungry are likely not going to be focused on what is healthy and good for you, be whatever you are craving at the time. By eating even a small snack before going shopping, you can prevent this from happening and stick with your list.

The time of day you go shopping also make a big difference in how long it takes to accomplish. Most grocery stores are busiest in the middle of the day or after work. The best time to go shopping is early in the morning right after breakfast. The store will be less crowded so you can be in and out in a flash and save yourself time.

You will have also just eaten, so you will be less likely to impulsively buy foods that are not on your list from being hungry. Later in the evening can also be a good time to shop if you are willing to go out then. Most people will be home by that point, so you will have most of the store to yourself.

Time-saving suggestions

Here are some tips and tricks that will make preparing meals a sustainable habit that you keep up with the long term:

- Use a single ingredient in multiple meals. This way you are having to chop and cook fewer things, cutting down the time you spend prepping your meals.

- Play music or your favorite movie or television show while working on your meals. Having something to entertain you will make the time seem like it flies by instead of dragging from boredom.

- Prepare larger amounts of a certain ingredient that you need in a week and freeze the rest. This works especially well for anything with a marinade because the extra time will give the flavor time to soak into the food as it is defrosting.

- This is also something you can do to regularly cut down the amount of time you spend preparing ingredients in a week. Your future self will thank you!

- If you have food that will take a long time to cook, start with that one first! This usually includes rice or potatoes. While that ingredient is cooking, you can work on preparing others that will not take as long. This way you will finish faster.

- Put labels on your meal containers. This is a good idea so that not only do you know what is in each container and what meal it is for, but you can also know when you cooked it. This will ensure that food does not stay in your refrigerator longer than it should.

- Have fun with your menu. By creating interesting ideas that play with words or planning a theme for your meals for the week, you can ensure you stay interested in what you're eating. This is also a good way to encourage yourself to try foods from different regions of the world or ones that you might not have thought of trying before.

- Have a consistent day where you prepare your meals. Choosing one day of the week that you will always prep meals on makes you more likely to stick with the plan and makes it easier to schedule the time to do it into your busy week.

- Know yourself. If you already know you don't like an ingredient or a type of food, then don't choose a recipe that includes it. Doing this makes you less likely to eat the meals you prepare and more likely to make unhealthy choices as a replacement. This defeats the purpose of prepping meals in the first place! Likewise, if you know you like an ingredient, then use it as much as possible in your menu.

Chapter Three

Breakfast Made Simple

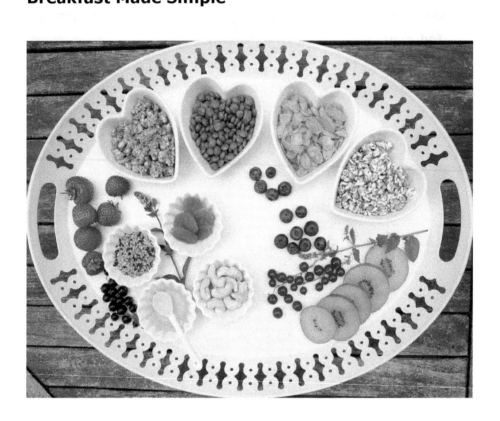

It's the most important meal of the day, so make it great.

Oatmeal while you sleep

What you will need

- Yogurt (.5 C)
- Milk (.25 C) – you can use almond milk to increase the amount of protein you are getting
- Cinnamon (a sprinkle)
- Nutmeg (a sprinkle)
- Vanilla flavoring (as much as you like)
- Traditional oatmeal (.5 C)

What to do

- Stir yogurt, cinnamon, nutmeg, and vanilla together
- Add in oatmeal to the mixture
- Pour in milk slowly until a good consistency is reached. You may decide to use a little more or less than recommended, depending on how thick you like your oatmeal
- Store in your refrigerator overnight. The oatmeal will soften in the yogurt mixture for a filling breakfast you don't have to spend a lot of time making

Make it yours

The toppings are where this recipe shines. The best combinations include fruit and nuts for a good balance of protein, healthy carbohydrates, and essential nutrients.

Whenever possible, choose seasonal fruits for a fresh, delightful breakfast. Use natural products, such as honey or maple syrup, to sweeten instead of sugar if you desire.

Flavor suggestions:

- Walnuts and pears
- Peanuts and bananas
- Hazelnuts and strawberries
- Macadamia nuts and pineapple
- Almonds and mandarin oranges
- Pecans and cherries

Make your freezer burritos
What you will need

- Cooked rice
- Eggs, scrambled (can be replaced with soft tofu)
- Tortillas (flour)
- Peppers and onions (one of each), sliced and sautéed
- Protein source (will depend on the theme)
- Fillings (will depend on the theme)

What to do

- Cook rice and let cool completely
- Cut up peppers and onions. Sautee in olive oil, then set aside to cool
- Cut and cook fillings and protein source (see below for details), then let cool
- Put your burritos together
  - Start by laying out a tortilla onto a cutting board
  - Then spread approximately .25 C of cooked rice in a line along the middle, leave space at both ends of the tortilla for folding
  - After this, spread approximately .25 C of scrambled eggs or tofu on top of the rice
  - Add a layer of sautéed peppers and onions on top of the scrambled eggs or tofu
  - Finally, spread protein and fillings on top of peppers and onions
  - Fold the top and bottom of the tortilla (the areas you left space while assembling the burrito) onto the fillings. Then fold one side onto the fillings and tuck around them. Finally, roll the burrito along the last side of the tortilla to complete

Make it yours

These burritos can be refrigerated to eat over a week, or they can be made in large batches and frozen to keep on hand for up to 3 months. They are easy to make in large batches, so freezing them is a perfect solution for long-term breakfast planning and will save you time in your meal prep. It is also very easy to use different flavors or themes in your burritos to keep breakfast interesting. Choose spices and seasonings that are appropriate to the theme you are working with.

Some suggestions:

- Mexican: black beans, corn, salsa
- Greek: chickpeas (also known as garbanzo beans), spinach, feta cheese
- Ethiopian: lentils, stewed tomatoes (make sure to drain well before using), cauliflower

French toast from the oven
What you will need

- Eggs (8 large)
- Milk (1 C)- you can use almond milk for an extra protein boost
- Cinnamon (1 tsp)
- Nutmeg (a sprinkle)
- Vanilla flavoring (1 tsp)
- Bread (about 12 slices or 1 loaf)

- Maple syrup (2 Tbsp)
- Fruit and nut fillings of your choice (about 2 C combined)

What to do

- Start by making sure your oven is set to heat to 375 degrees Fahrenheit.

- Then coat a glass cooking dish with oil to prevent your French toast from sticking. This is easiest if you use cooking spray.

- Prepare your eggs by putting them in a bowl and using a whisk to mix until thoroughly combined. Then combine in the cinnamon, nutmeg, vanilla, and milk while continuing to use the whisk. Set aside for later use.

- Tear your bread into bite-sized cubes. Try to get about 9 pieces per slice. Your French toast will be healthiest if you use whole grain bread instead of white bread.

- Take about half of your bread chunks and use them to create the first layer of your French toast in your glass cooking dish.

- Then take your fruit and nut mixture and spread about half of this on top of the first layer of bread.

- Finish creating your layers by adding the rest of the bread chunks followed by the rest of the fruit and nut mixture.

- Take the bowl containing the egg and milk mixture and spread this across the entire baking dish. Coat as much of the bread, fruit, and nuts as possible and try to avoid an uneven coating. If you want, sprinkle a bit more cinnamon and nutmeg on top after coating.

- Place your baking dish in the heated oven and set a timer for 35 minutes before checking to see if your French toast is done. Do this by taking a toothpick and inserting it into the middle of the dish. If it comes out clean, then it is finished! If not, cook for another 5 to 10 minutes at a time until the toothpick is clean.

Make it yours

Like with the oatmeal overnight, you can come up with endless flavor combinations for your French toast by trying different fruit and nut mixtures. You are only limited by your imagination and palate. You can use the same recommended flavors as for the oatmeal or try some new ones. Suggestions:

- Macadamia nuts, pineapple, and coconut
- Walnuts, raisins, and apples
- Pecans, persimmons, and plums
- Almonds, blueberries, and bananas

Muffin tin eggs

What you will need

- Cheese, shredded (cheddar is best)
- Tomato (1 large)
- Pepper (1 large)
- Onion (1 medium)
- Eggs (6 large)
- Spinach (1 bunch)
- Muffin liners

What to do

- Start by making sure your oven is set to heat to 400 degrees Fahrenheit.

- Take your spinach and remove all stems. Then roll leaves into a bundle (this makes them easier to cut) and slice into thin ribbons.

- After this, take your onion, pepper, and tomato and chop into small pieces. Combine these into a medium-sized mixing bowl with the spinach.

- Prepare your eggs by putting them in a bowl and using a whisk to mix until thoroughly combined. Add a sprinkle of salt to them to enhance their flavor.

- Combine the eggs with the chopped veggies and stir until everything is well blended and coated.

- Insert the muffin liners into a regular-sized muffin tin (usually makes 12 muffins). If you do not have muffin liners, then spray the tin with cooking oil so that your eggs don't stick to the sides during cooking.

- Spoon the vegetable and egg mixture into the muffin liners. Make sure you don't overfill or underfill any of the cups.

- Take the shredded cheese and add a little to the top of each cup.

- Put the muffin tin in the oven and set the timer for 15 minutes before checking to see if they are done. To do this, take your fingers and test the top of each egg cup. If they are firm, then they are done. If they are not done, put them back in the oven for 2 minutes at a time until they are firm

Make it yours

You don't have to stick to only one vegetable combination with these eggs. You can choose different themes and add appropriate vegetables to create new flavor combinations. However, when you are doing this make sure you are aware of how long the vegetables you are using take to cook. If they take a while (like potatoes), then you may need to precook them before adding to the muffin tins so that they do not come out hard by the time the eggs are finished.

Suggestions:

- Shredded carrots, green onions, zucchini
- Sweet potatoes, corn, and peas
- Butternut squash, green beans, and onions
- Green, red, yellow, and orange bell peppers
- Asparagus, chives, leeks, and potatoes

Make-ahead whole wheat pancakes

What you will need

- Milk (.6 C)- use almond milk for added protein
- Egg (1 large)
- Whole wheat flour (.3 C)
- White flour (.3 C)
- Cinnamon (a sprinkle)
- Toppings of your choice

What to do

- Separate egg yolks from whites. Set the yolks aside.

- Use a whisk to beat the egg whites until they are aerated. When this happens, they will be firm and produce peaks. Set aside.

- Combine cinnamon, whole wheat, and white flours using a sifter or fine-mesh strainer to avoid any lumps you may find.

- Add the egg yolks into the combined flours, stirring constantly. Slowly add the milk and stir well to prevent lumps from forming.

- Carefully add the egg whites into the flour mixture. You do not want to remove the air from them, so folding in with a spatula is the best way to do this.

- Set a stove burner to medium and place a small pan with a nonstick coating over the burner. Let it heat up until it is hot.

- Pour about .25 C of batter into the pan and let cook on one side.

- It is time to flip the pancake when you see bubbles come through the batter and create small holes. This means the first side is done the cooking.

- Flip the pancake to cook the other side. Be careful as you do this since you do not want to break the pancake or fold it over onto itself.

- Let the other side cook for several minutes. You can flip the pancake over again to see if it is done. When it is ready, it will be brown on both sides (but not too dark). After the first flip, it should be easy to flip again if either side needs to cook longer.

- Once they are cooled, you can freeze your pancakes for up to a month. To reheat, just pop in the toaster!

Make it yours

The toppings are where you can add some creativity to these pancakes. Top with yogurt, fresh berries, nuts, and a sprinkle of granola for a healthy, complete breakfast.

Conversely, you can create a savory pancake by using yogurt, granola, nuts, and shredded veggies such as carrots or zucchini. It is important to make sure you add nuts so that you are getting enough protein with your breakfast, but otherwise, the toppings are up to you!

Scrambled chickpeas with potatoes and crispy kale chips
What you will need

- Olive oil
- Potatoes (3-4 large)
- Onion (1 medium)
- Pepper (1 large)
- Chickpeas (1 can)
- Avocado (1 sliced)
- Kale (1 bunch)
- Feta cheese
- Garlic (2 cloves, diced)
- Salt (as much as you like)
- Pepper (as much as you like)
- Paprika (as much as you like)

What to do

- Take the potatoes (you can peel them or leave the peel on depending on what you like) and cut them into small cubes.

- Set a stove burner to medium and place a large pan over the burner. Let it heat up until it is hot.

- Add the olive oil to the pan and then add the potato cubes.

- Cook the potatoes until they have softened but are still slightly firm. Make sure you stir often so they do not stick to the pan or burn on one side.

- While the potatoes are cooking, chop the onion, pepper, and garlic.

- Once the potatoes start to soften, add the onions, peppers, and garlic. Continue to stir frequently.

- As the veggies are cooking, open the can of chickpeas and let most of the liquid drain out from them.

- Add the chickpeas to a bowl with the salt, pepper, and paprika. Use a fork to mash them all together. Don't mash too much, because this dish tastes better with chunks of chickpeas left with the mashed.

- Mix the chickpeas in with the potatoes and other veggies. Cook until the potatoes are soft enough that a fork goes all the way through them and remove from heat.

- Take the kale and tear from the stalks. Toss in a bowl with some olive oil and salt, pepper, and paprika.

- Place the kale on a baking sheet and put in an oven that has been heated to 425 degrees Fahrenheit.

- Set a timer for 8 minutes and take the kale out of the oven when it goes off. Stir it up on the baking sheet and place it back in the oven for another 5 minutes.

- When the kale is cooked, top a portion of the mashed chickpeas and potatoes with the kale chips. Add the feta cheese to the bowl as well.

- Cut the avocado into slices and add them to the bowl. It is best to do this right before you plan to eat it so that the avocado does not brown

Make it yours

Seasonings are where this recipe shines and stands out. You can change the flavor profile dramatically by changing which seasonings you use. This is a great place to experiment with regional flavors and spices. If you are portioning this out to eat over several days, do not add the kale until the morning you plan to have this for breakfast, otherwise, it will not stay crispy. Store the kale in an airtight container to retain its crunchiness.

Deconstructed smoothie in a bowl

What you will need

- Yogurt (2 Tbsp)
- Banana (1 medium)
- Fruit (1 C, frozen)
- Nut-based butter (2 Tbsp)
- Milk (2 Tbsp)- use almond milk for extra protein
- Granola
- Fresh fruit
- Chia seeds

What to do

- Using a blender, puree the frozen fruit and peeled banana until thick.

- Add the yogurt and nut-based butter and blend again. The mixture should be thick.

- Then add the milk to the blender and blend until it is a consistency you like. You may use a little more or a little less, depending on how thick you like your smoothie.

- Pour the smoothie into a bowl. Top your bowl with sliced fresh fruit, granola, and chia seeds

Make it yours

There is no end to the number of flavor combinations you can come up with for your smoothie bowls. You are only limited by what you can imagine. The key is to make sure that you use fresh and frozen fruits that go well together. Your smoothies can be stored in the fridge for up to a week or can be frozen after blended for up to a month. When storing, do not add the toppings until right before you plan on eating it for breakfast. This is especially true of the granola. If you refrigerate your smoothie bowls with the granola, it will become soggy and mushy.

Suggestions:

- Frozen mixed berries with slices of fresh strawberries and coconut.

- Frozen peach slices with fresh whole blueberries and banana slices.

- Frozen strawberries with fresh sliced mango and raspberries.

- Frozen tropical fruit with chunks of fresh pineapple and passion fruit.

- Frozen bananas with peanut butter, banana slices, and strawberries.

Chapter Four

Let's Do Lunch

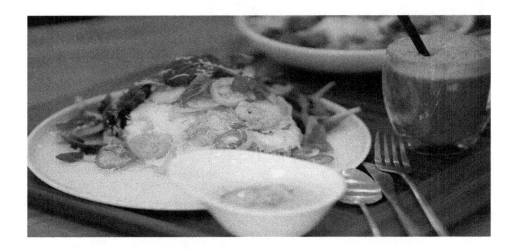

You won't even think about stopping at the drive-through with these fabulous lunch options.

Tuna replacement salad
What you will need

- Bread (sliced whole grain)
- Tomato (1 medium)
- Lettuce (several leaves)
- Celery (1 stalk)
- Mayonnaise (2 Tbsp)
- Chickpeas (1 can)
- Onion (1 medium red)

- Brown mustard (1 Tbsp)
- Pickle (1 large dill)
- Salt (as much as you like)
- Pepper (as much as you like)
- Garlic (1 clove, chopped)

What to do

- Take the celery, onion, and pickle and chop into fine pieces.

- Drain the water from the can of chickpeas, leaving a little bit in the can. Put the chickpeas into a bowl. Using a fork, mash them into a paste. This recipe tastes better and more closely.

- resembles tuna if you leave a few chunks of chickpea in the paste.

- Add the mayonnaise, brown mustard, salt, pepper, garlic, and any other seasonings you want to the smashed chickpeas. Mix until everything is combined completely.

- Combine the chickpea mixture with the chopped veggies and stir until everything is well blended.

- Refrigerate the tuna replacement salad for at least 1 hour until it is chilled.

- When you are ready to make lunch, slice up the tomato.

- Take a slice of the whole grain bread and layer it with the lettuce and tomato. If you want, you may want to add some extra sliced red onion and sliced pickles.

- Top the lettuce and veggies with approximately .25 C of the chilled, not tuna salad mixture and finish with the other slice of bread.

- This recipe can also make a great snack if eaten with vegetable slices or crackers.

- If you have the opportunity, you can make this lunch even better by taking time to toast the whole grain bread before you assemble your sandwich

Easy lunch burrito in a bowl

What you will need

- Olive oil
- Black beans (1 can)
- Corn (1 can)
- Salsa (3 Tbsp)
- Vegetable stock
- Quinoa
- Shredded cheese
- Avocado
- Cilantro (1 bunch)

What to do

- Start by cooking the quinoa. This is very similar to cooking rice. Measure out as much quinoa as you want into a large pot (2 C will make enough for a weeks' worth of lunches). Then add twice as much vegetable stock as quinoa to the pot. Cook the quinoa over medium heat until all the liquid has been absorbed and the quinoa is not hard.

- Take the can of black beans and drain the liquid from them. Then rinse them with water until the water is clear. Also, drain the corn at the same time.

- Set a burner on the stove to medium. Place a medium pan on the burner and heat until hot.

- Add the olive oil to the pan. Then add the black beans and corn. Season them with salt, pepper, garlic, and anything else you like. Cook until hot.

- Once the quinoa is cooked, add the black beans and corn. Stir them together until they are well mixed.

- When portioning out, top each lunch with a bit of shredded cheese, some cilantro, and the salsa.

- On the day you plan to eat this lunch, cut the avocado into slices and add them to the burrito in a bowl. Do not do this too early to prevent the avocado from turning brown.

Vegetarian lunch fajitas
What you will need

- Rice
- Vegetable stock
- Pepper (2 large)
- Onion (1 medium)
- Sweet potato (2 large)
- Garlic (2 cloves, chopped)

- Salt (as much as you like)
- Pepper (as much as you like)
- Cumin (a sprinkle)
- Chipotle pepper (.5 tsp)
- Paprika (1 tsp)
- Olive oil

What to do

- Start by making sure your oven is set to heat to 375 degrees Fahrenheit.

- Cook the rice. Measure out as much rice as you want into a large pot (2 C will make enough for a weeks' worth of lunches). Then add twice as much vegetable stock as rice to the pot. Cook the rice over medium heat until all the liquid has been absorbed and the rice is not hard.

- Peel the sweet potatoes and cut them into strips that resemble thin French fries.

- Place the sweet potato strips into a bowl with some olive oil. Add about half of the seasonings and coat the sweet potatoes with oil and spices.

- Pour the sweet potatoes onto a baking sheet and place your baking sheet in the heated oven. Set a timer for 10 minutes.

- While the sweet potatoes are baking, cut the peppers and onion into slices. It is best if you have two peppers of different colors.

- Places the peppers and onion into a bowl with some more olive oil. Add the other half of the seasonings and coat the peppers and onion with oil and spices.

- Pour the peppers and onions onto another baking sheet. When the timer has gone off for the first time, add this baking sheet to the oven with the sweet potatoes.

- Set the timer for 15 minutes. When it has gone off, take both baking sheets out of the oven and stir the vegetables. Place them back into the oven for another 15 minutes.

- For lunch, start with a bit of rice in a bowl and add the roasted veggies on top of it.

Turkish cannellini salad

What you will need

- Lemon (1, juiced)
- Olive oil (2 Tbsp)
- Salt (.5 tsp)
- White wine vinegar (1 tsp)
- Eggs (4, hard-boiled)
- Green onions (1 bunch)
- Cannellini beans (2 cans)
- Pepper (2 large)
- Dill (1 bunch)
- Cucumber (1 medium)
- Parsley (1 bunch)
- Tomato (1 large)

What to do

- Start by creating a dressing to go on the salad. Stir the vinegar, salt, olive oil, and lemon juice together. The best way to do this is with a whisk so that it will be thoroughly combined. Put this in the refrigerator to get cold.

  Take the peppers and chop them up into small pieces. They do the same thing for the tomato. Add both of these to a mixing bowl.

- Cut up the green onions, parsley, and dill until they are chopped finely. Add them to the bowl with the peppers and tomato.

- Open the cans of beans and let the liquid drain out from the cans. Wash the beans in water.

- Add the beans to the mixing bowl with the herbs and vegetables. Mix them until they are combined well.

- Take the dressing out of the refrigerator and use it to coat the bean and vegetable mixture. Make sure the dressing is evenly spread across everything.

- Slice the hard-boiled eggs into thin sections. Add a couple to each portion of the bean salad.

- This salad tastes good by itself, or you can eat it with crackers. It is also great spread across whole-grain toast slices.

Pocket salad sandwiches

What you will need

- Spinach (1 bunch)
- Tomato (1 large)
- Onion (1 medium red)
- Chickpeas (1 can)

- Cucumber (1 medium)
- Feta cheese
- Tahini dressing
- Lemon (1, juiced)
- Pita pockets

What to do

- Open the chickpeas and pour the water out of the can. Place these into a mixing bowl.

- Take the tomato, onion, and cucumber and chop into small chunks. Add these to the mixing bowl with the chickpeas.

- Coat the vegetables and chickpeas with the lemon juice. Mix them all in the mixing bowl to ensure they are all coated and well combined.

- Cut a pita and open each half up to reveal the pocket.

- Take the stems off the spinach. Line the pita on both sides with spinach.

- Fill the rest of the pita with the vegetable and chickpea mixture.

- Add some feta cheese to each pocket and drizzle with tahini.

Cucumber hummus rolls

What you will need

- Hummus
- Avocado (1 large)
- Cucumber (2 large)
- Tomatoes (1 jar, sun-dried)
- Garlic (1 clove, chopped)
- Basil (4 Tbsp)
- Salt (as much as you want)
- Pepper (as much as you want)
- Toothpicks

What to do

- Start by cutting the avocado in half and removing the pit. Spoon the contents out into a bowl and mash with a fork until creamy. Add the garlic and some salt and pepper. Cover and set aside in the refrigerator.

- Spoon the hummus out into another bowl. Add the basil and stir until well combined.

- Open the jar of tomatoes and let most of the juice pour out. Keep a little bit in the jar.

- Add the tomatoes and juice to the hummus. Stir again until combined well.

- Cut the ends off the cucumbers and slice long way into thin ribbons. This is easiest if you use a vegetable peeler or mandolin set to a thin slice.

- Lay the cucumber slices out. Spread a bit of the hummus mix onto each one. Then spread a bit of the mashed avocado on top of the hummus.

- Be gentle and roll the cucumbers up into spirals. Be very careful not to roll too tight and squeeze the fillings out as you are making your spirals. Skewer each spiral with a toothpick through both sides to keep them from unrolling before you have a chance to eat them.

Pasta-based garden salad
What you will need

- White wine vinegar (.5 C)
- Italian seasoning (2 Tbsp)
- Olive oil (.5 C)
- Garlic (1 clove, chopped)
- Salt (as much as you like)
- Pepper (as much as you like)
- Small tomatoes (1 package, cut in quarters)

- Corn (1 can)
- Pepper (1 large)
- White beans (1 can)
- Parsley (1 bunch)
- Tortellini (1 package)

What to do

- Heat a burner to high. Fill a large pot with water and set onto the stove. Add a sprinkle of salt and olive oil to the water and boil.

- As you are waiting for the water to heat up to boiling, mix the vinegar, salt, pepper, Italian seasoning, olive oil, and garlic. The best way to do this is to put everything into a jar and shake it until it is all completely combined. Set this in the refrigerator.

Cut the pepper up into small pieces. Put this in a mixing bowl with the tomato quarters. Open the can of corn and pour the water out. Add this to the bowl as well. Open the can of white beans. Pour out all the juice from the can. Wash the beans in a strainer before combining them in the bowl with the vegetables. Take the stems off the parsley and roll into a bundle for easy cutting. Slice this into small ribbons. Add to the vegetables and mix until combined well.

- Once the water boils, cook the tortellini. This should take between 5 to 8 minutes if it is fresh. If it is dried, this will take about 15 to 20 minutes.

- Once the tortellini are finished, place into a large strainer. Use cold running water to reduce the heat until cold.

- Place the tortellini into the bowl with the vegetables, beans, and parsley. Stir them all together until you have an even mixture.

- Take the dressing out of the refrigerator and use to coat the tortellini, beans, and vegetables. Mix thoroughly so that everything has an even layer of dressing on it.

- Refrigerate the salad until cold before eating for lunch.

Vegetable tortilla spirals
What you will need

- Mushrooms (1 package)
- Alfalfa sprouts (1 package)
- Carrots (2 large)
- Zucchini (2 large)
- Cucumber (1 medium)
- Onion (1 medium red)
- Pepper (1 large)

- Broccoli (1 head)
- Hummus
- Whole wheat tortillas
- Toothpicks

What to do

- Begin by cutting the onion into thin slices. Cut these in half so you have very thin onion strips.

- After this, slice the pepper into very thin strips as well. This recipe is best if you use a colored pepper. Then cut the cucumber into very thin round slices. This is easiest to do if you have a mandolin to use.

- Use a cheese grater to shred the carrots and zucchini. Make sure to remove all the water from both vegetables by squeezing over the sink. Then separate the squeezed clumps into piles of shredded vegetables.

- Cut the mushrooms up into small pieces. Do the same thing with the broccoli, focusing on the top parts. If you use the stem of the broccoli, make sure this is chopped very finely so that it does not tear up the tortillas or become too chunky to eat easily.

- Layout the tortillas. Take some of the hummus and use a knife to coat the tortilla evenly across the whole face.

- Sprinkle the alfalfa sprouts on top of the hummus. Ensure a good covering of the tortilla face.

- After this, sprinkle the onions, peppers, mushrooms, and broccoli on top of the alfalfa sprouts. Then layer this with the shredded carrots and zucchini.

- Finally, arrange the cucumber rounds across the tortilla face on top of the rest of the vegetables. Try to only overlap slightly and take care with how you arrange the rounds.

- Once this is finished, roll the tortilla into a spiral. Place 8 toothpicks evenly across the tortilla spiral so that they go all the way through. Cut the tortilla into spiral slices in between the toothpicks.

Jar salad constructions

What you will need

- Chopped vegetables (as many as you like- see suggestions)
- Nuts
- Grains
- Salad dressing
- Green leafy vegetables
- Protein source (beans, lentils, tofu)

What to do

- Start with a clean glass jar. Pour approximately 2 Tbsp of salad dressing into the bottom of the jar.

- Chop up your vegetables into small pieces. Separate these into crunchy vegetables and soft vegetables. Add the crunchy vegetables on top of the salad dressing in the jar.

- After this, add a layer of whatever protein source you are using on top of your crunchy vegetables.

- Place your grains on top of your protein source into another layer. It is okay if the layers end up mixing a bit. You will be eating it all anyhow!

- Then add your softer vegetables in a layer on top of your grains. Be careful not to pack these too tightly so that they get smashed up. You will want to combine any cheese you use with your softer vegetables.

- Your leafy green vegetables will go on top of your soft vegetables. Again, be very careful not to pack your jar too tightly. It will likely be getting full by this point!

- Finally top the jar off with your nuts, seeds, and other toppings before sealing and placing in the refrigerator until you are ready to eat it for lunch.

- Before you eat your jar salad, make sure the lid is tight on the jar. Then shake your salad enthusiastically to mix the dressing onto the contents and to hopefully mix the contents. This part will be a lot harder if you packed your jar tightly with food.

Suggestions:

- Mexican: chipotle ranch dressing, corn, peppers, black beans, quinoa, avocado, tomatoes, cheddar cheese, lettuce, tortilla strips.

- Sushi roll: wasabi soy dressing, shredded carrots, cucumber, edamame, rice, avocado, rocket, sesame seeds, almond slivers.

- Greek: Greek dressing, cucumber, red onion, chickpeas, orzo, tomato, olives, feta cheese, spinach, sunflower seeds.

- Middle Eastern: lemon Zaatar vinaigrette, onion, cucumber, radish, lentils, tomato, Romaine lettuce, chopped mint, pita strips.

Chapter Five

Daring Dinners

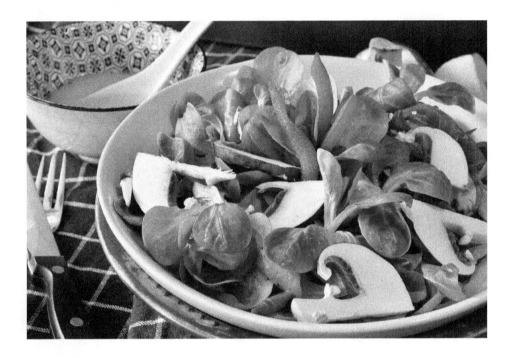

Why order takeout when you can wow yourself with quick and easy home-cooked meals?

Chinese style chickpeas

What you will need

- Rice, cooked
- Cornstarch (1 tsp)
- Brown mustard (1 tsp)
- Sesame oil (1 tsp)
- Chili sauce (2 tsp)
- Coconut sugar (4 tsp)
- Rice vinegar (1 Tbsp)
- Soy sauce (1 Tbsp)
- Creamy peanut butter (.5 Tbsp)
- Tomato paste (1.5 Tbsp)
- Vegetable stock (6 Tbsp)
- Chickpeas (1 can)
- Pepper (1 large)
- Broccoli (1 head)
- Onion (1 small)
- Olive oil (1 Tbsp)
- Garlic (2 cloves, chopped)
- Sesame seeds

What to do

- Start by cooking the rice. Measure out as much rice as you want into a large pot (2 C will make enough for a weeks' worth of dinners).

- Then add twice as much vegetable stock as rice to the pot. Cook the rice over medium heat until all the liquid has been absorbed and the rice is not hard.

- While the rice is cooking, you can start working on the sauce. Put the cornstarch, brown mustard, sesame oil, chili sauce, coconut sugar, rice vinegar, soy sauce, creamy peanut butter, tomato paste, and vegetable stock together in a bowl. Combine them until completely blended. The easiest way to do this is with a whisk.A Place to the side once combined.

- Cut up the onion, pepper, and broccoli into small pieces.

- Set a burner on the stove to medium. Place a large pan on the burner and heat until hot.

- Add the olive oil to the pan. Then combine with the garlic and onion pieces. Cook the onion until it becomes a little see-through. Make sure to mix often as the onion is cooking.

- Once the onion has cooked a little, combine the pepper and broccoli with it in the pan. Let them cook until the broccoli and peppers begin to be soft.

- Pour the sauce into the pan with the vegetables. Mix them until well combined and stir regularly while cooking.

- Open the can of chickpeas and pour out the liquid. Wash the chickpeas in a strainer after pouring out the liquid.

- Add the chickpeas to the pan and mix. Let the vegetables, chickpeas, and sauce cook until everything is hot.

- When serving or getting ready to store, place the rice in bowls or containers and put the vegetable and chickpea mixture on top. Sprinkle with some sesame seeds on top.

Squash-a-Roni and cheese
What you will need

- Cheddar cheese (1.5 C)
- Milk (.75 C)
- Vegetable stock (.5 C)
- Paprika (1 tsp)
- Butter (2 Tbsp)
- Butternut squash (3.5 C)
- Macaroni (1 box)

- Salt (as much as you want)
- Pepper (as much as you want)

What to do

- Make sure your oven is set to heat to 425 degrees Fahrenheit.

- Start by working on the butternut squash. Start by taking the peel off and removing both ends. Then cut it in half. Take the seeds out. The easiest way to do this is with a spoon. Chop the butternut squash into medium-sized cubes.

- After this, put the butternut squash into a mixing bowl. Add a little bit of olive oil and any seasonings you may want. Mix the squash and oil until it is even across the contents of the bowl.

- Pour the butternut squash onto a baking sheet. Put the baking sheet in the oven and set a timer for 30 minutes before checking to see if the squash is done. You can tell it is cooked when a fork goes all the way through it. If it is not ready, set the timer for another 5 minutes before checking again. Do this until it is cooked.

- Use a cheese grater to turn the cheese into ribbons.

- Heat a burner to high. Fill a large pot with water and set onto the stove. Add a sprinkle of salt and olive oil to the water and boil.

- While you are waiting for the water to heat, add the butternut squash, vegetable stock, milk, paprika, salt, and pepper into a food processor or blender. Puree until there are no lumps and everything is smooth.

- After the water has started to boil, you can cook the macaroni. This will take about 15 to 20 minutes. After it is done, place it in a strainer to remove the water.

- Set another burner on the stove to medium. Place a large pan on the burner and heat until hot.

- Put the butter in the pan and melt it. Then combine the macaroni in the pan with the butter and mix.

- Pour the butternut squash mixture into the pan with the pasta. Also, combine the cheese with the rest of the ingredients. Mix until everything is well combined and there is an even coat on all of the pasta. Keep the pan on the burner until the cheese is melted and everything is ready to serve.

Curried mixed vegetables

What you will need

- Rice, cooked
- Curry paste (2 tsp, whichever color you prefer)
- Maple syrup (1 Tbsp)
- Coconut milk (1 can)
- Vegetable stock (1 C)
- Onion (1 large)
- Frozen mixed vegetables (1 bag)
- Frozen peas (.5 C)
- Small corn (1 can)
- Ginger (2 tsp)
- Vegetable oil (2 Tbsp)

What to do

- Start by cooking the rice. Measure out as much rice as you want into a large pot (2 C will make enough for a weeks' worth of dinners). Then add twice as much vegetable stock as rice to the pot. Cook the rice over medium heat until all the liquid has been absorbed and the rice is not hard.

- Cut up the onion into small strips and place to the side.

- Set a burner on the stove to medium. Place a large pan on the burner and heat until hot.

- Put the vegetable oil in the pan with the ginger and onion. Cook the onion until it becomes a little see-through. Make sure to mix often as the onion is cooking.

- After this, you can combine the frozen vegetables with the onion in the pan. Cook for about 5 to 7 minutes.

- While the vegetables are heating you can open the can of small corn and pour the liquid out. Cut the corn into small chunks.

- Add the corn and peas to the vegetables and onion. Heat for another 5 minutes.

- Lower the heat on the stove burner before pouring in the coconut milk and vegetable stock. Cook until the liquid begins to bubble lightly. This should take around 10 to 15 minutes.

- Once the liquid is bubbling, combine the maple syrup and curry paste. Continue to let the mixture bubble lightly until it becomes slightly thick. Once it is thick, the curry is ready to serve.

- When serving or getting ready to store, portion the rice out into containers or bowls and add the curried vegetables on top.

- If you enjoy the taste, you can sprinkle some cashews or peanuts onto the curry to give it a bit of a crunchy texture.

Deconstructed lasagna bake
What you will need

- Pasta sauce (1 jar, either red or white- whichever you like better)
- Mozzarella cheese (2 C, shredded)
- Egg (1 large)
- Parmesan cheese (.5 C, grated)
- Ricotta cheese (1 container, 15 oz)
- Frozen spinach (1 package, 10 oz)
- Lasagna noodles (1 package)
- Salt (as much as you want)
- Pepper (as much as you want)

What to do

- Heat a burner to high. Fill a large pot with water and set onto the stove. Add a sprinkle of salt and olive oil to the water and boil.

- Make sure your oven is set to heat to 350 degrees Fahrenheit.

- Until the water heats, warm the spinach from frozen. You can do this by placing it in a bowl and heating in the microwave for 1 minute at a time.

Ensure all the water is removed from the spinach by squeezing it over the sink. Then separate the spinach clumps until you have a pile of warm spinach.

- Place the spinach into a mixing bowl. Mix in the egg, parmesan cheese, ricotta cheese, pepper, and salt. Combine until well mixed.

- After the water has started to boil, you can cook the lasagna. This will take about 15 to 20 minutes. After it is done, place it in a strainer to remove the water. Ensure the noodles are cooled by adding cold water from the tap into the strainer.

- Spread out the lasagna noodles. Place .3 C of the spinach combination on top of each noodle. Then roll the noodle into a spiral.

- Take a large glass baking dish and add 1 C of pasta sauce to the bottom. Be sure to coat it completely. Place the lasagna spirals into the baking dish with the end of the noodle at the bottom.

- Add more pasta sauce to the top of each spiral. Once they are covered, sprinkle the mozzarella cheese on top of the sauce.

- Cover the glass baking dish with a sheet of aluminum before putting it in the oven. Set a timer for 40 minutes before checking to make sure they are done. You will tell this because the cheese will be melted and slightly golden.

- When serving or getting ready to store, coat the bottom of each plate or container with a little bit more pasta sauce before adding the lasagna spiral.

Stewed Spanish-style chickpeas with spinach
What you will need

- Rice, cooked
- Spinach (2 bunches)
- Chickpeas (1 can)
- Tomato paste (1 Tbsp)
- Tomatoes, canned (2 cans, 28 oz)
- Brown sugar (2 tsp)
- Onion (1 medium red)
- Salt (as much as you want)
- Paprika (1.5 tsp)
- Powdered hot pepper (.25 tsp- you can add more if you like spicy food)
- Cumin (3 tsp)
- Garlic (3 cloves, chopped)
- Olive oil (2 Tbsp)
- Sliced almonds (.25 C)

What to do

- Start by cooking the rice. Measure out as much rice as you want into a large pot (2 C will make enough for a weeks' worth of dinners). Then add twice as much vegetable stock as rice to the pot. Cook the rice over medium heat until all the liquid has been absorbed and the rice is not hard.

- Cut up the onion into small strips and place to the side.

- Set a burner on the stove to medium. Place a large pan on the burner and heat until hot.

- Put the olive oil in the pan with the garlic and onion. Cook the onion until it becomes a little see-through. Make sure to mix often as the onion is cooking.

- Mix the paprika, powdered hot pepper, cumin, and salt into the onion and garlic combination. You can leave the powdered hot pepper out of the recipe if you do not like spicy food. If you do this, then increase the amount of paprika and cumin by .5 tsp each to retain enough flavor. Continue to heat and stir regularly
- Combine the tomato paste into the pan and heat until it starts to thin slightly.

- Open the can of tomatoes and smash them with their liquid still combined. This is easiest if you pour them into a bowl and use a potato masher. Combine them into the rest of the ingredients with the sugar in the pan. Let the mixture cook until lightly bubbling. Make sure you mix it up from time to time so that nothing sticks to the pan.

- Once the tomato stock has turned slightly thick, open the can of chickpeas. Pour the liquid out and wash the chickpeas before mixing them into the pan. Heat until the chickpeas are hot.

- Finally, remove the stems from the spinach. Add the leaves of spinach to the pan and add a lid to it. Let the mixture heat until the spinach is no longer firm. This should take about 5 to 10 minutes.

- When you are ready to serve or store, place some rice in the bottom of the bowl or container you are using. Put some of the stewed chickpeas on top of this. Finally, sprinkle with the almond slices.

Spicy vegetable Cajun stew
What you will need

- Rice, cooked
- Parsley (1 bunch)
- Cilantro (1 bunch)

- Paprika (1 Tbsp)
- Thyme (2 tsp)
- Cajun seasoning (2 Tbsp)
- Powdered hot pepper (2 tsp)- you can leave this out if you do not like spicy food
- Tomatoes (1 can dice)
- Zucchini (1 medium)
- Kidney beans (1 can)
- Mushrooms (1 package)
- Celery (2 stalks)
- Pepper (2 large)
- Onion (1 medium red)
- Okra (12-15 pieces)
- Olive oil (.25 C)
- Flour (.25 C)
- Liquid smoke
- Worcestershire sauce (make sure to check the ingredients label to find a vegetarian version)
- Salt (as much as you want)
- Pepper (as much as you want)

What to do

- Start by cooking the rice. Measure out as much rice as you want into a large pot (2 C will make enough for a weeks' worth of dinners). Then add twice as much vegetable stock as rice to the pot. Cook the rice over medium heat until all the liquid has been absorbed and the rice is not hard.

- Then cut the mushrooms, peppers (this recipe tastes best if you use two different colors), zucchini, celery, okra, and onion into small pieces.

- Set a burner on the stove to medium. Place a large pan on the burner and heat until hot.

- Put the olive oil in the pan and heat until very hot and ready to bubble when other ingredients are added. Then add the flour in small amounts at a time and combine well. The best way to do this is with a whisk. Keep adding flour and mixing until you have combined all of it with the oil. Continue to mix and let the flour and oil for about 8 to 10 minutes until it turns brown to create a roux. Be very careful not to let this burn.

- Pour the vegetable pieces into the pan. Combine the vegetables and roux with the liquid smoke and Worcestershire sauce. Heat the vegetables for approximately 10 minutes until they are no longer hard.

- Sprinkle the vegetables with the paprika, powdered hot pepper, thyme, Cajun seasoning, salt, and pepper. Then remove the stems from the parsley and cilantro and roll them into a bundle. Cut them into thin slices and add to the vegetables as well.

- Open the can of kidney beans and pour out all the liquid. Wash the beans in a strainer until the water you are using becomes clear.

- Pour the kidney beans into the vegetable mixture. Open the can of tomatoes and pour out a little bit of the liquid but keep some of it. Add this to the pan also.

- Let the mixture of vegetables, beans, and tomatoes heat until the tomato stock becomes slightly thick. This should take approximately 20 minutes.

- When you are ready to serve or store, place some rice in the bottom of the bowl or container you are using. Then add some of the Cajun stew on top of this. You can sprinkle with a bit more of the fresh parsley and cilantro if you like the taste to accentuate the flavor.

Chapter Six

Snack Attack

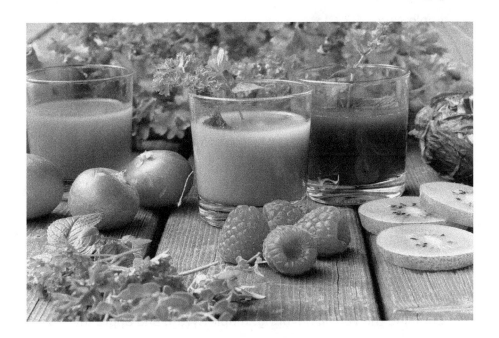

Catch those cravings before they hit!

Oatmeal pizza with fruit
What you will need

- Fruit mixture (2 C)
- Oatmeal (3 C)
- Cinnamon (1 Tbsp)
- Eggs (2 large)

- Vanilla flavoring (1 tsp)
- Maple syrup (.5 C)
- Salt (.5 tsp)
- Apple sauce (.3 C)
- Greek yogurt (2 C)

What to do

- Make sure your oven is set to heat to 375 degrees Fahrenheit.

- Take a glass pie dish and coat it with spray oil to prevent sticking.

- Place salt, cinnamon, and oatmeal into a large mixing bowl. Stir to make sure it is all well mixed.

- Combine the vanilla flavoring, maple syrup, and apple sauce with the eggs. Mix until well combined. The easiest way to do this is with a whisk.

- Create a hole in the middle of the cinnamon, salt, and oatmeal combination to pour the egg, applesauce, vanilla, and maple syrup combination into. Mix them until well combined and there are no dry, flaky spots or lumpy areas.

- Pour the bowl contents into the glass pie dish. Use the back part of a spoon or your fingers to pat the mixture down until it is firm and holds together.

- Put the dish into the oven and set a timer for 10 minutes before checking to see if it is cooked. You will know this when the mixture is a little brown but not too dark. If it is not done, set the timer for another 2 minutes at a time before checking again.

- Once the pie dish comes out of the oven, place it onto a wire rack to let heat dissipate. Leave it there and set a timer for 10 minutes.

- Once the timer goes off, take the oatmeal mixture out of the glass pie dish and set it back onto the wire rack to let more heat dissipate. You need to leave it there until it is not hot at all anymore. You can make this happen faster by putting the entire rack into the refrigerator and set a timer for about 10 minutes.

- Once the base is not hot anymore, pour the yogurt onto it. Use the back of a spoon to push it evenly around the entire surface.

- After you have added the yogurt to the base, put it back into the refrigerator for an hour or longer so that it becomes cold and starts to keep its shape.

- Once the yogurt is cold, cut up any fruit that needs to be cut. If it does not need to be cut, like blueberries or raspberries, you can leave it complete. Make sure to use as many of your favorite fruits as possible to make this pizza taste great.

Decoratively put the fruit on top of the yogurt. Try to make sure that each slice will have a little bit of all the different fruits you use.

- Use a knife to make separate slices of your pizza. If you want, you can add dollops of whipped cream on top of each piece for an extra treat.

Sweet and spiced pumpkin cupcakes

What you will need

- Coconut oil (3 Tbsp, melted)
- Eggs (2 large)
- Vanilla flavoring (1 tsp)
- Whole wheat flour (3 C)
- Maple syrup (.5 C)
- Milk (1 C)- use almond milk for an added protein boost
- Salt (.75 tsp)
- Baking soda (1.5 tsp)
- Pureed pumpkin (1 C)
- Cloves (a sprinkle)
- Nutmeg (.25 tsp)
- Cinnamon (1 Tbsp)
- Ginger (1 tsp)
- Allspice (a sprinkle)
- Muffin liners

What to do

- Make sure your oven is set to heat to 375 degrees Fahrenheit.

- Insert the muffin liners into a regular-sized muffin tin (usually makes 12 muffins). If you do not have muffin liners, then spray the tin with cooking oil so that your cupcakes don't stick to the sides during cooking.

- Put the cinnamon, allspice, ginger, nutmeg, cloves, baking soda, salt, and whole wheat flour into a bowl. Combine until well mixed. The easiest way to do this is with a whisk.

- Put the pureed pumpkin, maple syrup, coconut oil, vanilla flavoring, milk, and eggs into a different bowl. Combine until these are well mixed also.

- Pour the flour combination into the milk combination and mix until there are no lumps and all the ingredients are completely mixed. Be careful not to stir too much. This will make your cupcakes tough and not taste as good.

- Pour the combination into the muffin cups. Try to make sure that each cup has an even amount of mixture in and that some are not too full or not full enough. If you think you would like the taste, you can sprinkle a little bit of coconut sugar on the top of each muffin cup.

- Put the tin into the oven and set a timer for 15 minutes before checking to see if they are cooked. Do this by taking a toothpick and inserting it into the middle of the dish. If it comes out clean, then it is finished! If not, cook for another 3 minutes at a time until the toothpick is clean.

- When the cupcakes are cooked, take them out of the oven and put the pan on top of a wire rack to dissipate heat. Set a timer for 5 minutes. Once the timer has gone off, take the cupcakes out of the pan and put them back on top of the wire rack until they are not hot anymore.

Once there is no heat left in your cupcakes, you can keep them fresh in the refrigerator for a week. If you want to make a lot of these at once, you can put some of them in the freezer. They can stay frozen for 3 months before they are no longer good.

Make your healthy whole wheat and grain bread
What you will need

- Oatmeal (2 Tbsp)
- Sunflower seeds (2 Tbsp)
- Salt (.5 Tbsp)
- Whole wheat flour (2 C)
- Water (1.5 C, warm)
- Yeast (.75 Tbsp, or 1 envelope)
- Maple syrup (2 Tbsp)

- Salt (.5 Tbsp)
- White flour (1.75 C)

What to do

- Use a big mixing bowl to add the maple syrup, water, salt, whole wheat flour, yeast, and white flour. Mix these ingredients until well combined. The result will be very sticky and coarse. When a spoon is no longer strong enough to move through the sticky mixture, use your hands to continue combining inside the bowl.

- As you are combining the ingredients with your hands add extra flour until it does not stick to you or the bowl anymore. Do this by mixing in .5 C at a time and alternate between white flour and whole wheat flour.

- Spray another bowl with cooking oil so that your bread batter doesn't stick to the sides. Move the batter from the first bowl into the new bowl that has been sprayed with oil. Add a sheet of plastic to the top of the bowl and leave it on the counter so that the batter can get bigger. You want it to be two times as big as when you put it in the bowl.

Once the batter has become big, open a hole in the middle of it to put the oatmeal and sunflower seeds into. Sprinkle flour onto your kitchen counter and move the batter from the bowl to the counter.

Mix the batter by hand again until it is stretchy and bounces back a little bit. This will take you around 20 minutes to accomplish.

- Once your batter is stretchy and the oatmeal and sunflower seeds are well spread out throughout the entire mixture, use your hands to create a round shape with it.

- Spray a baking sheet with cooking oil so that your bread batter doesn't stick to it while it is cooking. Move the shaped batter from the counter to the baking sheet and sprinkle a little bit of flour on the top. Cover it with another sheet of plastic and set a timer for 45 minutes before checking to see if it has gotten bigger again. You want the shaped batter to be twice as big as when you put it in the baking sheet. If it is not, set the timer for another 15 minutes before checking again.

- While you are waiting for your batter to get bigger, make sure your oven is set to heat to 425 degrees Fahrenheit.

- Before you put the baking sheet in the oven, cut the shaped batter with a knife in a diagonal pattern 3 times. Only cut about .5 deep and be careful not to cut too far into the batter.

- Put the baking sheet in the oven and set a timer for 25 minutes before checking to see if it is done. You will know this when the entire shape is light brown but not too dark.

You can also test whether or not your bread is done by lifting the shaped batter and tapping the bottom of it with your fingers. A hollow-sounding knock means it is cooked in the middle.

- When the bread is cooked, take it out of the oven and put the baking sheet on top of a wire rack to dissipate heat. Set a timer for 5 minutes. Once the timer has gone off, take the bread off of the baking sheet and put it back on top of the wire rack until it is not hot anymore.

- Once there is no heat left in your bread, you can keep it fresh in the refrigerator for a week. If you want to make more than one bread at once, you can put some of them in the freezer. They can stay frozen for 3 months before they are no longer good.

- Your bread will be perfect for so many uses in your healthy diet. You can create fantastic sandwiches, tasty toasts, or eat it on its own with a little bit of honey or nut-based butter. This is a recipe that can do anything!

Cookies that are good for you
What you will need

- Egg (1 large)
- Salt (.5 tsp)
- Baking powder (1.5 tsp)
- Honey (.5 C)

- Oatmeal (1 C)
- Cinnamon (1.5 tsp)
- Vanilla flavoring (1 tsp)
- Whole wheat flour (.75 C)
- Any nuts, flavored chips, or other ingredients you want to mix in (.5 C)

What to do

- Make sure your oven is set to heat to 375 degrees Fahrenheit.

- Spray a baking sheet with cooking oil so that your cookies don't stick to it while they are cooking.

- Use a big bowl to combine the cinnamon, baking powder, whole wheat flour, salt, and oatmeal. Mix until well combined. The best way to do this is with a whisk.

- Heat the butter until it is melted. Pour this into a different bowl with the honey, egg, and vanilla flavoring. Mix these until well combined, also using the whisk.

- Pour the butter mixture into the oatmeal mixture and combine with a spoon. Mix until there are no lumps and all the ingredients are completely mixed. Be careful not to stir too much. This will make your cookies tough and not taste as good.

- Pour your nuts, chips, or other ingredients into the mixture and combine until they are completely mixed in and even in the entire batter.

- Move the bowl to the refrigerator and set a timer for 30 minutes before taking it back out.

- Form your cookies into balls using your hands. You should be able to create about 15 balls with one single recipe. You can easily make more at a single time if you want without needing to use a lot of extra effort to do so. If you do this. You can separate the batter into different types of cookies and add different fillings to each batter.

- Arrange the batter balls onto the baking sheet. Make sure to leave space in between them so that they do not run together while cooking. 2 inches should be enough to prevent this.

- Put the baking sheet into the oven and set a timer for 12 minutes before checking to see if they are done. You will know this when the sides of the cookies at the bottom are a little brown but not too much. If they are not cooked, set a timer for 2 minutes at a time until they are.

- When the cookies are cooked, take them out of the oven and put the baking sheet on top of a wire rack to dissipate heat. Set a timer for 5 minutes.

Once the timer has gone off, take the cookies off of the baking sheet and put them back on top of the wire rack until they are not hot anymore. If you want. You can add more fillings to the top of the cookies as soon as you take the baking sheet out of the oven.

Crunchy chickpeas in the oven

What you will need

- Your favorite spice flavor(s) (4 tsp)
- Chickpeas (1 can)
- Salt (1 tsp)
- Olive oil (2 Tbsp)

What to do

- Make sure your oven is set to heat to 425 degrees Fahrenheit.

- Open the chickpeas and pour the liquid out of the can. Wash the chickpeas in a strainer until the water is clear.

- Set out two sets of paper towels that have been layered. Pour the chickpeas onto one set and cover with the other. Rub vigorously to remove all the water from washing. If any shells have come off during this, you can throw them away.

- Pour the chickpeas into a mixing bowl. Combine with the salt and olive oil. Blend until well combined and the chickpeas all have oil covering them completely. If you want, you can add a little bit of your spice flavor into the mixture before cooking. If you do this, make sure you save the listed amount for later as well.

- Pour the chickpeas onto a baking sheet. Move them around to make sure they are not clumped up in one area and are spread across the entire baking sheet so that they cook evenly.

- Put the baking sheet in the oven and set a timer for 10 minutes. When the timer goes off, take the baking sheet out of the oven and move the chickpeas around on it. This will prevent only one side from cooking and make sure they bake evenly all around their entire surface.

- Once you have moved the chickpeas around, put the baking sheet back in the oven and set the timer for another 10 minutes before doing the last step over again. You will want to do this 3 times before taking the baking sheet out of the oven for the last time when the chickpeas are finished cooking. You will know they are done when they are dark brown all over but not black and all of the oil has been cooked off. They will feel soft inside but be crunchy outside.

- Once the chickpeas are cooked, pour them into a mixing bowl with your favorite seasoning. Blend the chickpeas and spices until well combined and the chickpeas all have spices covering them completely.

- These crunchy chickpeas are great by themselves as a snack instead of eating potato chips or something else unhealthy. You can also add them to lunches or dinners to add extra flavor and crunchiness to whatever you are eating. They are never a bad addition since they are good to get protein from and can increase this in any meal.

Conclusion

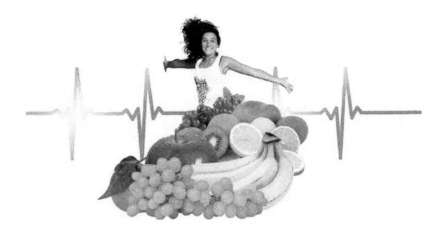

I hope you enjoyed your copy of Vegetarian Meal Prepping:

The Exclusive Guide for Ready-to-Go Meals for a Healthy Plant-Based Whole Foods Diet with a 30-Day Time- and Money-Saving Easy Meal Plan. Let's hope it was informative and provided you with the tools and knowledge you need to get started prepping healthy vegetarian meals all week.

The next step is for you to start implementing what you learned from this book into your diet! Your time and money are valuable, so save both of them by using this guide to start prepping your meals once a week instead of cooking every day, or even worse- going back to the drive-through!

Start by deciding which type of meal prep described inside you want to start with and is the best fit for you. Then schedule when you will make time to go grocery shopping and when you will prepare your meals. From there, choose your favorite recipes from this book to get started with and create your menu. Keep in mind which fruits and vegetables are currently in season for the freshest possible options. Then make your grocery list and go shopping. Finally, get started with prepping your meals! As long as you stick to this easy to follow the guide, you can make meal prep and a vegetarian diet a sustainable lifestyle that takes little to no effort to keep up with!

If you found this book useful in any way, a five star review is always appreciated !

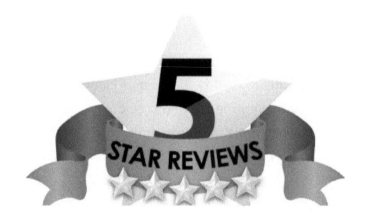

ALL RIGHTS RESERVED. This book contains material protected under International and Federal Copyright Laws and Treaties. Any unauthorized reprint or use of this material is prohibited. No part of this book may be reproduced or transmitted in any form or by any means, electronic or mechanical, including photocopying, recording, or by any information storage and retrieval system without express written permission from the author/publisher.

The author is not a licensed practitioner, physician, or medical professional and offers no medical diagnoses, treatments, suggestions, or counseling. The information presented herein has not been evaluated by the U.S. Food and Drug Administration, and it is not intended to diagnose, treat, cure, or prevent any disease. Full medical clearance from a licensed physician should be obtained before beginning or modifying any diet, exercise, or lifestyle program, and physicians should be informed of all nutritional changes.

The author/owner claims no responsibility to any person or entity for any liability, loss, or damage caused or alleged to be caused directly or indirectly as a result of the use, application, or interpretation of the information presented herein.

Vegan Meal Prep

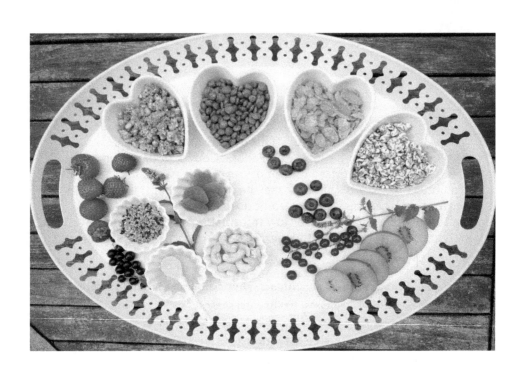

The Ultimate Book For Ready-To-Go Meals For a Healthy, Plant-Based, Whole Foods Diet With 4 Weeks Time And Money Saving, Easy And Quick Meal Plan.

104

Description

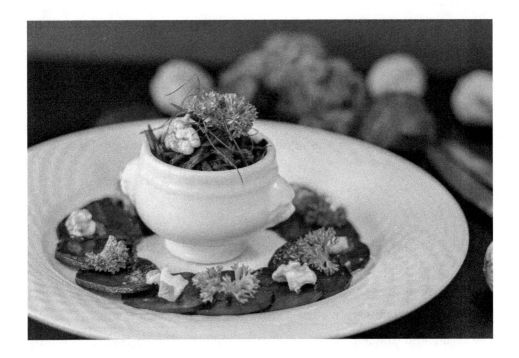

If you are looking for great ways to save money and at the same time eat healthy meals every day of the week, then this meal prep is your perfect companion. At times, preparing vegan meals may seem complicated and overwhelming. Fortunately, this list of vegan meal prep ideas will not only help you to prepare easy meals, but they will also be delicious.

It does not matter even if you are just starting on a vegan diet or you just want to try it out and see how it goes.

Whichever your case, the point is that meal prep offers an amazing option to ensure you have healthy meals throughout the week.

The benefits you gain from <u>Vegan Meal Prep</u> are quite encouraging. They give you the morale to do more. When you do meal prepping, you are guaranteed more time during the week to do other stuff.

You will not be pushed to create time from crazy schedules to go shopping. In fact, your shopping times will become fewer, less hectic and shorter.

Vegan meal prep will save you the worries of what to cook every day. As much as you may be creative with your meals, there are those times your mind is just blank, and this can be very stressful. However, if you practice meal prepping, that can never be your portion. It helps you to know what exactly you intend to make for breakfast, lunch, dinner, desserts, and snacks. As a result, you will be able to feed on healthy and nutritious meals every eating time without straining.

Would you love to prepare vegan for cheap?

It is the desire of every person to eat healthy and tasty food. The recipes and ideas in this book will help you meet your desires.

Is it possible to prepare your meals for 5 days in advance?

Yes. However, make sure you keep the meals in the refrigerator.

Are you on a diet and wants to learn how to prepare vegan meals for weight loss?

If you are on a diet or are planning to do so to lose weight, then vegan food can help you do just that. With a vegan diet, you will be able to replace unhealthy meals with foods low in calories and keep fuller longer.

Do you want to learn how to meal prep for a week of vegan lunches?

Perfect. This book entails all you need to know in regards to preparing healthy meals to take you the whole week.

The beauty of this book is that it contains informations that are beneficial to you and your loved ones.

You do not have to feed on junk and unhealthy meals just because time is not on your side. Whether you are a student or a committed worker, vegan meal prep allows you to prepare healthy meals for the whole week.

In this easy meal prep, you will learn the easiest way to prepare all your meals in super easy ways. You will have healthy and delicious vegan meals for you and your loved ones to feed on.

Why you need to read this awesome book

- This book is the only place you will learn how to prepare healthiest meals.

- The book is suitable for people of all walks of life.

- Assist students who need ready meals on the go.

- Enable busy parents to feed their families with healthy meals.

- Help you significantly reduce food wastage.

- If you are not the type who loves to cook every other day, you are well sorted with **vegan meal prep**.

- It will help you to save time, money and still feed on delicious healthy meals.

- The recipes are suitable for both adults and children.

- You will learn how you can prepare delicious meals even on a budget... and more...

Table of Contents

Bonus tips for making healthy desserts super tasty

Consider these tips;

Use seasonal fruits

Make it with nuts

Use real sweeteners

Use high-quality ingredients

Chocolate chip gingerbread

Healthy no bake cherry vegan cheesecake

Making the No-Bake Cherry Cheesecake

Vegan matcha coconut tarts

Doughy peach pie bars

No-bake blueberry custard pie (vegan and gluten-free)

Banana chocolate and peanut butter swirl bread with pecan praline

Dark chocolate almond oatmeal cookies with sea salt

3-ingredient guilt free brownies

Creamy lime and avocado tart

Vegan brown rice crispy treats

Chapter 4: Snack meal prepping

Healthy meal prep snacks

Chapter 5: Vegan meal prep high protein

Easy vegan chili sin carne

High protein salad

Mexican lentil soup

Black bean and quinoa balls

Chapter 6: Vegan meal prep weight loss

Tips to lose weight as a vegan

Conclusion

Introduction

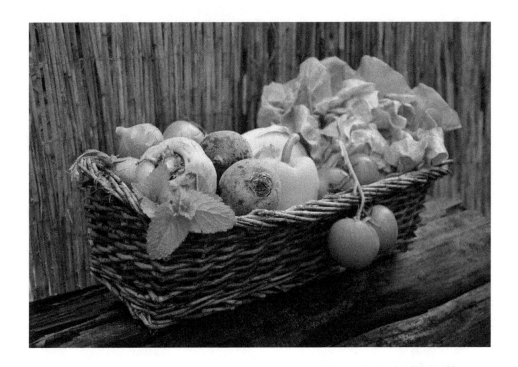

Congratulations on buying Book *"**Vegan Meal Prep"**,* and thank you for doing so.

The following chapters will discuss how it is possible to eat healthy even when you are short on time. By being equipped this book all your meal prep will be budget-friendly, and you'll have assistance to stick to your diet, even when you have a busy week.

There are several books on this subject, thanks for choosing this book.

We made every effort to ensure that every piece of information is of use and importance to you, our reader. Please enjoy!

How to get started

What is vegan meal prepping?

Before you get started, it is better to understand what vegan meal prepping entails so that you will have an easy time when preparing these healthy meals. Vegan meal prep is about cooking some healthy meals ahead of time and then portioning them out throughout your week.

First of all, you begin by planning what you intend to eat and then prepare a grocery list based on the recipe you chose. This way, you will save time, money, and at the same time, feed on much healthier meals throughout the week.

Best tips for meal prepping

In everything you do, some basic guidelines go a long way, and vegan meal prep is not an exemption. Therefore, below are some important tips to help you start your vegan meal prep accordingly. Why is this important? It will help you to know the meals to cook in advance. You will also learn the best way to keep your food fresh for the longest time possible. There are also some equipment suggestions. All these are done to give you an easy time when preparing your meals.

Healthy, safety and storage tips

a) High protein foods

You need to be extra careful when it comes to high-protein foods. While plant-based foods tend to have a much lower risk or chance of food poisoning, it will still pose a certain level of risk.

The reason as to why foods high in protein need to be well taken care of is because bacteria tend to thrive more on food with high protein content in comparison to starches and sugars. For instance, it is advisable you take extra care when storing and reheating foods like rice and quinoa to eliminate any chances of food poisoning.

b) Fridge or freezer?

Any food you choose to store in the fridge should be consumed within 2 to 3 days. Hence, if you are not sure that you will have consumed some meals within that duration, then it is safe to store it in the freezer. Simply, remember to get it out of the freezer and maybe now put it in the fridge a day before the day you intend to have it.

c) Your Senses

Fortunately, your senses can help you decide if you can consume a certain meal or not. By using your sense of smell or sight, you can be able to determine whether the meal is safe to consume.

Note that tasting the meals to see if it is safe to eat is the last thing you should do if you care about your health.

d) Reheat properly

You do not have to be in so much hurry when reheating your food least you end consuming something that will lead to your next hospital visit. Make sure you thoroughly reheat your foods and consume them when they are still hot. On top of that, always ensure that you keep cold meals at lower temperatures and hot meals at higher temperatures. You should avoid keeping hot and cold meals at room temperature. According to the USDA, bacteria are more likely to thrive in temperature between 4 and 60 degrees Celsius. How do you tell your food is hot enough? Make sure you note some hot piping in the middle of reheated meals.

e) Do not put warm food in the fridge

When you decide to keep warm meals in your fridge, chances are the food will affect the fridge's overall internal temperature. This may put the other foods in the fridge at risk of spoiling. To avoid this, always ensure that the meal cools off first before placing it inside the freezer or fridge.

f) Defrost timely

As mentioned above, refrigerated meals should be consumed within 2 to 3 days. Frozen meals should be fully defrosted in the fridge or at room temperature before you even think of consuming them. Always remember this when preparing your meals for the entire week.

Suitable storage equipment to consider

Here are some awesome options for storing meals you prepared earlier. Plastic food containers. When choosing a plastic container, go for the ones that are safe to use in the microwave and dishwashing machine. Boxes/Glass Jars. If you do not prefer using plastic to store your food, then glass jars present a perfect choice. This should be your number one option for all your basic storage options. Ziploc-style bags. You can use Ziploc-style bags in your freezer or fridge. They are also economical since you can use them multiple times. Lunch boxes offer a perfect storage option, especially if you are storing the meals in portions to easily grab as you head out. You can also use them if you want to keep different foods separately.

What to consider when choosing a recipe

One amazing factor about meal prepping that you can enjoy a good number of delicacies throughout the week even when you have a lot to do in your workplace or school so long as you took your time to prep in the start of the week. To help you get the most out of your experience with vegan meal preps, below are some awesome ideas to guide you. No worries, you don't have to grab everything. The point is, even if you fail to get the hang of things right away, with time, you will be able to tell what works for you and what does not. You will also be able to know the perfect portions for you at each meal time.

115

Begin with your favorite foods

In the beginning, go for recipes that contain foods you had eaten before and enjoyed. If you are not ready to try a new recipe or food combo, then ensure that all ingredients are paired with things familiar to you.

Plan out your recipe

Planning out your recipe is something you should never fail to do if you want to prepare meals you will enjoy eating for the whole week. Start by visualizing what you intend to prepare the day before you go for your shopping. Have a list of the foods you need to buy to avoid getting confused at the grocery store. This will also help you to reduce impulse buying, whereby you may buy foods that will not be eaten and end up going to waste.

Get to know the best ways to combine foods

Ideally, a good but simple meal prep combo has legumes, starches, vegetables/greens, and condiments.

Make your own condiments

Do you love salads? Then why not consider making dressings and sauces ahead of time and keep them in the refrigerator? They can even go up for a whole week. By doing this, you are going to be able to add any type of raw veggie salad to your ideal legume or grain. Then add your pre-prep dressing.

Frozen Produce

The impressive feature of frozen fruits and vegetables is that they are affordable, fresh, and usually pack a lot of nutrients with them. It is also possible to refrigerate them for a longer time, and even when you need to prepare them; you will not have a hard time doing so. This is because any trimming or chopping needed has already been done for you. The best foods to buy frozen are things such as berries, mangoes, cherries, broccoli, peas, cauliflower, and root veggies, including butternut and squash.

Chapter 1: Vegan breakfast meal prepping

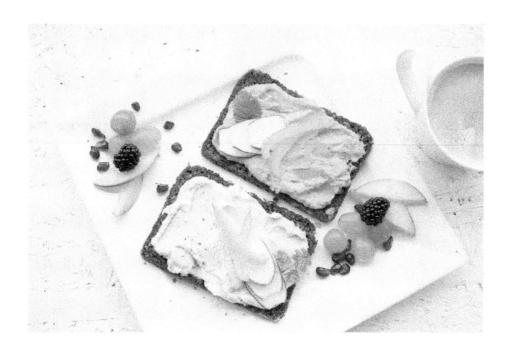

Who does not love starting their day with some delicious breakfast? Whether you like your breakfast salty or sweet, this chapter has got your back. The truth be told, breakfast can be a bit tricky, especially to plant-based people. Oatmeal or smoothie recipes offer a great option, but this can get a little bit boring, especially if this has become your everyday meal.

There are those crazy mornings when you don't have time to apply makeup or even dry your hair. Cooking a full meal is not on the list, and healthy eating can easily feel like the last thing you want to consider while it is crucial to your overall health.

Good news, the power to solve this nightmare is in your hands, simply consider planning. If you do so, you will be able to prepare delicious meals that you can stock in the freezer and simply grab on your way out. Isn't that amazing?

Below are delicious recipes you can prepare ahead of time to enable you to have a healthy breakfast even when you are rushing out. They are not boring and not just that, they will make your mornings brighter.

1. **Vegan zucchini bread**

If you like it dense and moist and you do not want to add butter, the secret would be applesauce. You will love the results. The bread also freezes well. The perfect way to enjoy a full serving of veggies without realizing it is by treating yourself with this comforting baked treat. If you like, you can whisk up a mixture of sugar, cinnamon and coconut oil/butter and spread it on top.

2. **Berry beet acai bowl**

Try this earthy veggie with some tart berries and coconut flakes. Sure enough, you will want some more. This meal is not only sweet but also full of vitamins. Simply blend your beets with acai, mixed berries, and coconut milk.

If you want to have it at its best, prepare it at night, and then store it in the fridge overnight so that the following morning you will just enjoy your delicacy as you head out. You can add your favorite toppings like hemp seeds and fresh berries, and the results will be something that is enough to brighten up your mornings.

3. **Freezer oatmeal cups**

No easier way to enjoy some oatmeal if not in this meal-prep hack. Cook enough of your morning oats, pour them into muffin tins and freeze them until they become solidified. In the morning, when you are ready to eat, simply get one of your frozen oats, put them on a bowl and microwave them. If you want to add more taste, just add your favorite milk and toppings of choice, and there is your awesome breakfast.

4. **Vegan potato and bacon**

Gone are days when special treats were left for the weekend and holidays when you have all the time you need to prepare your breakfast. You can also enjoy a tasty meal for your busy weekday mornings as well. This recipe provides you with an impressive solution. Here, you will need a diced potato, tofu, and vegan bacon. Wrap them in a flour tortilla. Alternatively, you can also try corn if you want it to be gluten-free. Although it is tempting to overstuff it, make sure you leave enough space to wrap if effectively for storage. In the morning, if time is on your side then take advantage of that and top with salsa and avocado.

5. Vegan freezer burritos

Seems like an awkward choice for breakfast? The good thing about this type of meal is that you can have it for breakfast and still enjoy it at any other time of the day. The good thing about burritos is that they are freeze enough to store for the longest time possible. Try this, your burritos, tofu scramble, roasted potatoes, veggies, steamed kales, beans, vegan cheese and anything else you would love to add. For instance, if you are eating the burritos fresh, avocado or guacamole does miracles. Overall, this meal is just tasty.

6. Peanut butter green smoothie freezer packs

This is what you do. Choose when you have time, maybe during the weekend, mix those ingredients and put them in the fridge. There are no rules here you can customize them just the way you like. Remember to subdivide them into portions before storing them. This will make things easier when you want to have some in the morning before heading out. When you are ready to use them, take one of the portions and blend it. If you are running out of time, put it in a portable cup, and you can have it on your way.

7. Banana quinoa breakfast

This option of breakfast is perfect for people with a sweet tooth. It will help them lead a healthy lifestyle. Another impressive thing about the banana quinoa breakfast is that it is naturally filling due to the fiber and protein in quinoa and nut butter. For that little extra crunch, add some coconut flakes.

8. Banana breakfast cookies

If you want to have granola in portable form, then consider this type of cookies. They consist of a combination of oats, chia seeds, and banana. To prepare it, whip the whole butch in about 30 minutes. You can then freeze it and then in the morning or whenever you want to enjoy this wonderful meal, microwave it. If you want them to be more filling, consider spreading some jam, coconut yogurt or nut butter on top.

9. Baked hash browns

Hash browns offer one of the best greasy brunch foods. They are not only crispy, but they are also carby. Those little slices are quite appetizing. If you want, runny egg or some zesty hot sauces do wonder. You do not need the sketchy oils they are normally fried in to make these hash browns. Just remember to freeze before you bake them. With this healthy meal in the freezer, you have no reason to leave the house in the morning with an empty stomach. You will need to pop them in the oven and if in not so much hurry, top with avocado.

Chapter 2: Vegan lunch and dinner meal prep

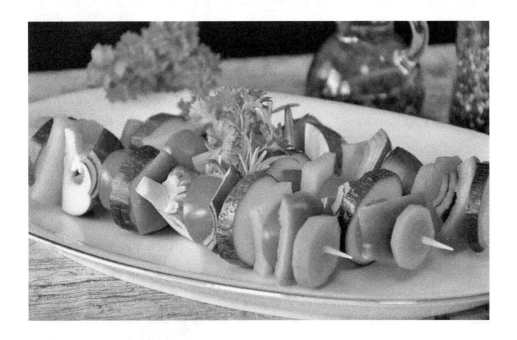

In this chapter, the book will guide you through super-simple ways to create delicious vegan lunches for a whole week. Incorporating a vegan diet or eating more plant-based meals has a lot of benefits to your overall health.

Healthy vegan meals will help you lower your risk of contracting diabetes, heart disease, and cancer. Furthermore, you have higher chances of reducing weight or even maintaining a healthy weight because those filling fiber foods such as veggies, fruits, whole grains, and beans will ensure you are satisfied when you consume them.

Lunch and dinners are the most laborious meals of the day. You might be tempted to snack out unhealthy meals, especially if you are having a busy week. Thanks to the vegan meal prep ideas, you can make those meals a bit easier without compromising their quality.

Just a little meal prep goes a long way. You have the power to make lunch or dinner something everybody wants to have a share in by just some simple planning, slicing and dicing, and just a few strategic sauces. More so, even if these recipes are vegan, it will surprise you how tasty they can be.

Below is a prep plan to help you prepare healthy meals for the whole week. Interestingly, these tastier recipes will ensure you have an easy time throughout the week and still feed yourself and your loved ones healthy, tasty meals. They will thank you later. You may be required to adjust the recipes depending on the number of people you are preparing the meals for. Do not worry, if you happen to realize what you made is excess, then how about you use the leftovers to dinner this week?

Enjoy healthy, delicious and easy to make meals. By the end of this, you will have become a pro to all matters regarding vegan meal preps.

Orange tofu chickpea bowls

This is one of the healthiest and delicious meal prep for lunch. They also come in handy for a quick and easy weekday dinner.

The orange tofu chickpea bowls are easy to make, full of flavor and filling as well. They offer a great option as a meal prep lunch that you can enjoy throughout the week.

Do you feel like this is something you would love to give a trial? Well, simply cook up the tofu and chickpeas, steam the broccoli, cook your rice and mix up the sauce.

You can use white rice for your grain, but you can still opt for other choices such as your favorite grain or cauliflower rice. The idea is to use your favorite or what you already have on your hands. The same case, if you do not want to use broccoli, you can use other substitutes like sugar snap peas, carrots, asparagus and the like. If you like your sauce thicker, then cook it a bit longer but bear in mind that it will be lesser. In other words, the lighter it is, the more you will get.

If you are making for meal prep, then get good sized portions and put them in the freezer. It would be better to heat them before eating to avoid any issues of food poisoning.

How to prepare it:

Measure your ingredients depending on the number of people you intend to prepare the meals for.

What you will need;

- Rice or your favorite grain
- Broccoli
- Extra firm tofu (cubed)
- Sesame oil or cooking oil of your choice
- Low sodium tamari
- Optional toppings such as sesame seeds and sliced green onions

Orange sauce;

- Freshly squeezed orange juice
- Low sodium tamari
- Toasted sesame oil
- Pure maple syrup
- Grated garlic
- Grated fresh ginger
- Cornstarch

Preparation

Cook your rice the way you like or follow the package directions. Steam the broccoli to your desired tenderness.

Use a small bowl or jar to add all the orange sauce ingredients. Mix them thoroughly and ensure they are well combined.

Add some oil and heat a large skillet. Keep the heat at medium. Then add tamari, tofu and then sauté the connection until the tofu turns brown. Occasional stirring in about 7 to 10 minutes is recommended.

Then add your chickpeas and orange sauce to the pan. Allow them to cook until the sauce becomes thick enough to coat your cooking spoon. The longer it cooks, the thicker the sauce becomes. So, if you want to have more sauce, do not allow it to cook for too long.

In each bowl, add some rice, broccoli, orange tofu, and chickpeas. If there is extra sauce available, drizzle it over rice and broccoli. Then season it with some soy sauce.

For meal preps, divide the meal into ideal portions, put them in the refrigerator/microwave safe containers and store them in the fridge. You can keep them up to 5 days. Make sure you properly heat them in the microwave or on the stovetop before eating them.

Chickpea and lentil taco salad meal prep bowls

This meal prep plan of chickpea and lentil taco salad meal prep bowls are healthy, tasty and filling.

What you will need to prepare this awesome meal. Measure depending on the number of people and the days you intend to serve this meal.

- Olive oil or your favorite oil
- Cooked chickpeas
- Cooked lentils
- Ground cumin
- Garlic powder
- Paprika
- Salt
- Corn kernels
- Onion powder
- Mixed greens or chopped lettuce
- Diced tomatoes
- Diced red onion
- Optional toppings like salsa, jalapenos, cilantro or black olives

For crispy tortilla stripes;

- Corn tortillas
- Cooking spray
- Salt
- Paprika
- Garlic powder

Greek yogurt ranch;

- Greek yogurt or any other non-dairy yogurt
- Diced cucumber
- Chopped basil

- Chopped Dill
- Chopped green onion or chives
- Garlic powder
- Onion powder
- Salt

Instructions to prepare

Begin by preheating your gas or electric oven to around 375 degrees F. place the thinly sliced strips of tortillas and place them on a medium sized sheet pan. Use the cooking spray to spray and season with garlic powder, paprika, and salt to taste. In about 7 to 10 minutes, it should have become crispy and starting to turn brown. Allow them to cool and then separate them into equal portions. Put them in a Ziploc bag or airtight container and store them on the counter.

Get a blender, put all the dressing ingredients inside and blend them until they become creamy. Put your dressing into different containers in equal amounts and then refrigerate them.

Next, heat a huge skillet. Keep the heat at medium. Then add your favorite oil, lentils, chickpeas, and all the remaining spices. Stir until the mixture combines and allow it to cook until it is heated through for the spices to develop. This should happen in about five minutes.

Now, get your choice of prep containers and in each of the container add some chickpea/lentil mixture, corn, lettuce, tomatoes, and red onion. Whenever you are ready to eat, you can top with dressing, crispy tortilla strips or your favorite topping and enjoy your lunch and dinner throughout the week.

Curried chickpea salad meal prep bowls

If you are looking for super easy healthy meal prep for lunch or at times dinner, then these curried chickpea salad meal prep bowls have the solution you seek. Interestingly, they do not require cooking, and you can be able to prepare them in 20 minutes.

Curried chickpea salad is just amazing and can make you look forward to your lunches the whole week so long as you know you will enjoy eating such a hearty salad.

The sweetness of incorporating curry in your diet is the great flavor it comes with. It also really goes well with apples, dried cranberries and of course chickpeas. For those lunches, you just don't want to feel fuller and tired, opt for this salad for a perfect light lunch option.

There are times when no-cook meals come really in handy. They provide the easiest and quickest way to make a tasty salad. They are also healthy as they are prepared with lots of fresh ingredients.

Although they are a favorite to many all year round, they tend to be more popular during summertime when everybody is avoiding heating their homes by turning the oven on. If you want to separate your crackers and grapes/mixed nuts from the chickpea salad, simply use separate containers or store your salad in a plastic bag.

It is advisable you add your crackers and mixed nuts when you are about to have your meals. If you put them earlier, they might become a little bit soft on the third and fourth day. So, if you like to keep everything crispy and fresh, you know what to do. If you do not want to have lettuce, feel free to exclude them. You can just scoop your curried chickpea salad with crackers and still enjoy your salad. You can include any fruits or sides of your choice such as grapes and mixed nuts, and you will be good to go.

What you will need

- Cans chickpeas, rinsed and drained
- Diced celery
- Diced apple
- Chopped red onion
- Dried cranberries
- Vegan mayo
- Dijon mustard
- Curry powder
- Salt
- Black pepper

- Lettuce
- Crackers
- Grapes or mixed nuts

How to prepare the salad

Add the chickpeas to a small bowl and slightly mash them using either a fork or a potato masher. Then add all the other remaining ingredients in the same bowl and mix them until they are super combined. After that, line up your meal prep containers. Add a lettuce leaf and the chickpea salad mixture to all your containers depending with the portion you like. You can separate the crackers and grapes/mixed nuts with some liners if you want.

Roasted Brussels sprout and chickpea meal prep bowls

What a healthy meal is full of vegetables and protein! You can make this awesome meal ahead of time and enjoy it later over lunch or dinner. Quite convenient, right?

Roasting chickpeas makes them so crispy and spicy too. Although they tend to loose a bit of their crispiness once they are refrigerated, then still come out nicely when warmed up. What about roasting vegetables? Superb. Roasting veggies brings their perfect flavor even before adding any spices.

Some helpful tips to consider:

Instead of dressing the bowls and you are not yet ready to eat, it is better to store the dressing in another container.

When it comes to avocado, add it in the morning to avoid it turning brown. On the same note, squeezing a little lemon juice over it can help prevent browning.

You can enjoy these bowls, either cold or warm.

Things you will need:

- Uncooked quinoa
- Brussels sprouts
- Cooked chickpeas
- Olive oil
- Garlic powder
- Salt
- Paprika
- Dried cranberries
- Black pepper
- Avocado

Lemon tahini dressing:

- Tahini
- Lemon juice
- Salt
- Warm water

How to prepare it

Switch on the oven and preheat the oven to around 400 degrees F. Follow the instructions on the quinoa packaging, cook and set it aside.

Rinse the Brussels sprouts, cut off the stem, peel off the out leaves if you like and slice it in half. Get a large sheet pan and add the sliced Brussels sprouts and chickpeas.

Drizzle everything with some olive oil. Then season with pepper and salt. To the chickpeas, add the paprika and garlic powder. Toss each ingredient gently until all is well coated. Bake them until the Brussels sprout becomes tender and turns brown. The chickpeas should also be crispy. This should take about 30 to 40 minutes. For the dressing ingredients, add them in a small bowl or a jar. Whisk them until they combine properly. You can put the dressing inside an airtight container until ready to use it. Your meal is now ready. Assemble your bowls. Make sure each bowl contains quinoa, Brussels sprout, and chickpeas. On top of that, add some dried cranberries. For the avocado, consider adding it when ready to eat.

Roasted summer vegetable meal prep bowls

This is another meal filled with delicious summer vegetables. Make this healthy, filling and delicious meal at the start of the week and enjoy a whole amazing week of ready lunch or dinner.

If you like, you can leave your cherry tomatoes raw. However, you should try roasting them and enjoy the sweetness that comes with it. The good thing about these roasted summer vegetable meal prep bowls is that they can be enjoyed either warm or cold.

If you are not able to find fresh basil, then consider using parsley. Top it with a store-bought balsamic dressing or whatever kind of dressing you like and make things easy for you.

What you will need:

Get the ingredients depending on the portions you intend to make and the number of days you will be enjoying this delicious meal.

- Diced zucchini
- Diced summer squash
- Pint cherry tomatoes
- Diced red onion
- Olive oil or your favorite cooking oil
- Salt
- Pepper

- Dried Italian seasoning
- Rinsed quinoa
- Chickpeas
- Optional fresh herbs for garnish
- Balsamic dressing (homemade or store-bought)

How to prepare

Begin by pre-heating the oven to around 400 degrees F. Get a large baking sheet enough to hold the diced zucchini, summer squash, onion and cherry tomatoes. Pour some olive oil and then season with salt, Italian seasoning, and pepper. Make sure the vegetables are evenly coated. Then roast for about 30 minutes or until tender and then start to caramelize.

Add quinoa in a pot and cover it with some cold water. Bring them to a simmer. Make sure that quinoa if well cooked with no more water. About 12 to 15 minutes should be enough. After it's ready, set it aside.

Using safe refrigerator containers, assemble the meal prep bowls. In each bowl, ensure you add some quinoa, chickpeas and the roasted veggies.

Once through, top the meal with fresh herbs and balsamic dressing. No restrictions here, even your dressing of choice will be perfect.

The bowls can be refrigerated for up to four days. If you are re-heating these bowls, ensure that they are microwave/oven safe.

Easy Greek salad meal prep bowls

These super easy Greek salad meal prep bowls are not only flavorful, but they are also loaded with tons of healthy vegetables. If you are looking some healthy vegan meal prep recipes, this should on top of the list.

The good thing about this recipe is that it provides such a fresh and flavorful dish. In fact, it gives you a perfect excuse to eat all the veggies on your plate. You simply need a few extra minutes to meal prep these easy Greek salad prep bowls. They are a life saver. Just make them on Sunday, and you will have lunch and dinner ready for the next 3 to 4 days of that busy week.

If you love fresh tomatoes, peppers, and cucumbers, then do not fail to put them on your Greek salad meal prep bowls for that perfect sweet taste they bring. No worries, if these are not your perfect choices, then feel free to use your favorite vegetables.

Do you feel like using chickpeas and hummus in the same dish a bit redundant? Well, this should not be the case because the textures are a little different, and on top of that, it is never a bad idea to have more proteins. Just experiment with using different hummus flavors and you will love the results.

You can also serve this meal prep with some toasted pita bread cubes. It is good for your carbs. Further, it acts like a crouton and gives your salad a nice texture. Only add the pita bread when you are ready to eat because if you add it earlier, it might get soggy.

What you will need

- Your favorite greens such as romaine, spinach, baby kales and the like
- Diced cherry tomatoes
- Diced bell pepper
- Diced cucumber
- Kalamata olives
- Cooked chickpeas
- Hummus
- Pita bread
- Olive oil
- Salt
- Dried Italian seasoning

How to prepare

Start by preheating the oven to around 350 degrees F to make pita bread croutons. If you like, you can dice pita bread into bite-size pieces. Use a large baking sheet to toss together the pita bread with a drizzle of olive oil and salt. Add Italian seasoning to taste. Then bake the pita until it turns brown and crispy, flip it once.

It should be ready in about 5 to 7 minutes. Store your pita croutons in an airtight container on the counter for no more than 4 days.

In each bowl, put a handful of greens, chickpeas, tomatoes, cucumber, bell pepper, kalamata olives, red onion, and hummus. Make sure you put them in airtight containers and refrigerate them for 3 to 4 days. If you happened to use a delicate green such as spring mix, then it is better you store it separately since it may not be able to hold up with all the other vegetables. When ready to eat and then top it with your favorite dressing and enjoy.

Sheet pan tofu and vegetable bowls with ginger peanut sauce

The idea of sheet pan meals comes really in handy, especially when you don't have enough time to clean every single dish in the kitchen. You can prepare this awesome meal and still leave your kitchen in good order. Basically, a sheet pan meals entail cooking the entire meal on a sheet pan in the oven. If washing dishes is not your thing, you will fall in love with this idea and end up doing it more often. If you want, you can add some rice but it is certainly not a must.

These sheet pan tofu and vegetable bowls offer a perfect healthy weeknight dial or meal prep lunch to be enjoyed by all family members.

What you will need (depending with the portions you intend to make)

- A packet of extra firm tofu
- Toasted sesame oil
- Tamari or soy sauce
- Garlic powder
- Diced red pepper
- Diced carrots
- Broccoli florets
- Snap peas
- Diced yellow onion
- Salt
- Ground ginger
- Black pepper
- Optional white rice or quinoa
- Optional garnishes

Ginger peanut sauce

- Creamy peanut butter
- Water
- Toasted sesame oil
- Tamari or soy sauce
- Pure maple syrup
- Rice wine vinegar
- Finely grated garlic
- Sriracha
- Salt

How to prepare

Pre-heat the oven to 400 degrees F. Then, drain any excess water from the tofu. Use a dish towel to press it for not less than 15 minutes if you can be able to press it for longer, the better.

After that, cut the tofu into bite-sized cubes, and then add them into a bowl. In the same bowl, add some sesame oil, tamari and garlic powder. Mix them properly and let the mixture settle for about 10 minutes or so. In a sheet pan with non-stick mat, add all the vegetables. Toss the vegetables with sesame oil, garlic powder, ginger, salt, and pepper. Move the vegetables to one end of the pan to leave enough space for the tofu. Then dump the tofu onto the pan along with any other extra marinade.

Bake the tofu and vegetables for about 35-40 minutes. The tofu should turn brown while the vegetables should be tender. Remember to flip once. While this is going on, save time by making the peanut sauce. Simply add all ingredients to a bowl and whisk until combined.

Your dish is now ready. Assemble the bowls and in each of them add your favorite grain to the bottom of the bowl, top with vegetable mix and the tofu. Drizzle the desired amount of ginger peanut sauce on top. Then garnish with your choice of garnishes and enjoy.

Vegetarian Mason jar burrito bowls

The beauty about vegetarian Mason jar burrito bowls is that they are healthy, full of flavor and easy to assemble. They also provide an impressive make-ahead lunch for all family members.

Although it is not a must you enjoy this meal from a mason jar, this makes it super easy to store and portion your burrito bowls. It will be easier to take them off during meals time.

What you will need

- Dried white or brown rice
- Diced sweet potatoes
- Drained and rinsed black beans
- Corn kernels
- Salsa/Pico de gallo
- Olive oil
- Salt
- Pepper
- Chopped cilantro
- Lime juice
- Guacamole
- Lettuce

How to prepare it

Pre-heat the oven to 375 degrees Fahrenheit. Take the chopped sweet potato and toss with some olive oil, a pinch of salt and pepper. Bake the sweet potato for about 35 to 40 minutes or until fork tender.

Cook the rice the way you like it or better still follow the directions on the package. When rice is ready, stir in the chopped cilantro and lime juice.

In the assembled burrito bowls, put some rice, black beans, sweet potato, corn, salsa, a spoonful of guacamole and some lettuce. For best results, when you are making these burrito bowls ahead of time, consider leaving out the lettuce and guacamole until when you are ready to serve. If you intend to heat the burrito bowls warm, simply stick the Mason jar in the microwave for about 1 minute. Once warmed, add in the lettuce and guacamole and enjoy this tasty meal.

Tex-Mex sweet potato lunch bowls

There are those days you just feel tired for no apparent reason. Even when you think you have taken a long night rest, you still wake up feeling tired. It is on such days you want to grab the easiest and most convenient thing to eat. In that case, a perfect option would be Tex-Mex sweet potato lunch bowls. Come to think of it, why would you not spend an hour or so making some Tex-Mex sweet potato lunch bowls and end up eating a healthy and filling lunch all week long?

That would be amazing, and there will be no room to unhealthy snack foodstuff. You will always look forward to lunch time every single day of the week.

These bowls are perfect for people who struggle to eat healthy lunch every day or someone who feels like time is not on their side when it comes to preparing a healthy, tasty meal. In that case, simply make them on Sunday and the following week will be a special one to you and your loved one.

What you will need

- Sweet potatoes
- Dried quinoa
- Drained and rinsed black beans

Avocado dressing:

- Pitted avocado
- Juice of 2 limes
- Minced garlic
- Salt
- Ground cumin
- Black pepper
- Water

How to prepare it

Begin preparation by pre-heating your oven to around 4oo degrees Fahrenheit's. Line a medium-sized baking sheet with foil or parchment paper. Use a fork to pierce each of the sweet potatoes a few times until they become fork tender. This should take you about 45 to 50 minutes.

Cook the quinoa in your liking or according to the directions on the package. In a blender, put all the dressing ingredients and then blend the mixture until it becomes creamy. 30 seconds to 1 minute should be enough. Your meal is ready.

Then assemble the lunch bowls. Cut the sweet potato open, top with quinoa and black beans. Drizzle your desired amount of dressing on top and if you like, serve with greens and chips. If you are not ready to serve, then leave the dressing and any other additional toppings until when the times comes to enjoy your tasty meal.

Spiralized sweet potato enchilada bowls

If you want a make-ahead lunch or some quick dinner, the solution would be these delicious sweet potato enchilada bowls. If you do not have a spiralizer, no worries, these sweet potato enchilada bowls can also be made with grated sweet potato instead of spiralized. However, if you are in for a spiralizer, simply make then thin enough to cook pretty quickly in a frying pan. Your dinner will be ready in less than an hour.

Making recipes that double as quick and easy dinners and meal prep lunch are never a bad idea. These sweet potato enchilada bowls are just like that. They are perfect for a family dinner or make ahead lunches for a whole week. Alternatively, you can have some for dinner and the leftovers for lunch. Either way, you will have still enjoyed this Mexican food to the fullest.

What you will need

- Olive oil
- Diced yellow onion
- Diced red pepper
- Diced green pepper
- Pilled and spiralized sweet potato
- Corn kernels
- Rinsed and drained black beans
- Cumin
- Paprika
- Granulated garlic
- Salt
- Enchilada sauce
- Optional rice or quinoa
- Optional toppings such as diced avocado, tomato, cilantro or salsa

How to make it

Switch on the heat to medium heat. Then add the olive oil and onion. Sautee the onion for about 2 minutes and then add peppers and sweet potato. Cook the veggies until tender, but it should not go beyond 10 minutes least you spoil your delicacy.

Add the black beans, corn, and all the spices. Stir and allow to cook for about two minutes. Then pour enchilada sauce and mix until well combined. Cook for about 5 minutes to ensure everything is well heated.

If you like, you can serve over rice and top with your favorite toppings. If you are making them as meal prep lunch, portion the enchilada mixture into the desired portions and pair with rice or quinoa.

Chapter 3: Dessert meal prepping

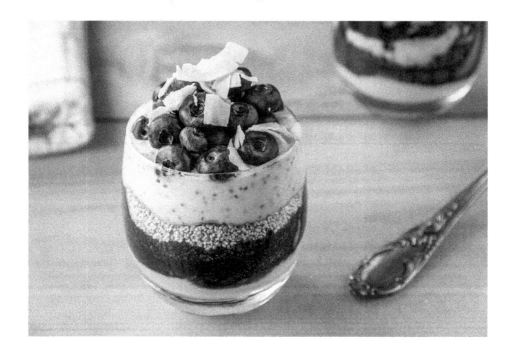

You can still satisfy your sweet tooth without compromising your clean, healthy lifestyle if you are equipped with healthy dessert ideas. Funny enough, most people are afraid to embrace clean eating simply because they fear the change will stop them from enjoying their foods anymore.

As much as some certain sacrifices have to be made to lead a healthy lifestyle, it's never easy to let go off your favorite meals. Saying goodbye to desserts is even more challenging. Life without holiday desserts, birthday cakes, and all the sweet treats must sound horrible.

Fortunately, you do not have to go through all those nightmares in the name of eating healthy. You simply need to go for the real, whole ingredients and adjust your favorite recipe just a little bit. When it comes to desserts, things are not different, either.

Now, do you want to learn how to make healthy desserts? Perfect. In this chapter, you will come across the best tips you need and some delicious totes recipes you will love. They also include so many healthy alternatives such as light desserts, low-fat desserts, low-calorie desserts, quick healthy desserts and easy healthy desserts all in one chapter. After this, you will forget about stressful dessert time.

Now that you have your meal prep lunch and dinner ready, it is your high time you add another course to your weekly prepping sessions. What could that be if not the below mentioned desserts? They are super easy to make, totally tasty and better yet, they are sweeter than you can imagine.

Helpful toolset for easy healthy dessert recipes

To ease up things much further, here is a list of tools that you can use to make some easy healthy desserts for your loved ones.

Mixing bowls: You need this for sure. They are somehow mandatory in any kitchen. As much as you will need them for your healthy desserts, they are still useful for other types of foods. Hence, the more reason you need to invest in nice mixing bowls.

A loaf pan: This is another kitchen essential you need to own. It has many uses, but for this particular case, you will be using it for ice cream, slices of bread, bars, and cheesecakes.

Mixer: are you ready for some healthy desserts recipes? Well, if yes, then make sure your mixer is ready as well.

Kitchen blender and food processor: Still in the same topic of kitchen gadgets to help you make super healthy desserts, you will need these two kitchen gadgets.

A trimmed baking sheet: This one will allow you to freeze fruits, turn them into the sorbet and make baked goods.

Cookie sheet/cooling sheet: Who does not love cookies? You will need a cookie sheet when you bake those delicious cookies and a cooling rack for cooling them.

Popsicle mold: A popsicle mold will come in handy when making those numerous healthy popsicle recipes. Do not hesitate to try them out.

Bonus tips for making healthy desserts super tasty

Great news! Numerous desserts can be made healthy. Therefore, forget about those misleading ideas that unhealthy desserts taste less than the healthy ones. The truth is, healthy desserts are very tasty. Just try the recipes below, and you will agree with this statement.

Consider these tips;

Use seasonal fruits

There is no doubt to this, seasonal fruits taste better and hence make a notable difference in your dessert. Consider using them in your dessert recipes as often as possible.

Make it with nuts

Nuts can make your dessert taste better. You can even replace the classic base with a nut-base for healthier desserts. You surely need to make your desserts with nuts not unless you have a nut allergy.

Use real sweeteners

Some healthy desserts become unpopular because they are not sweet enough. People with a sweet tooth feel the difference, and that is understandable. To change this scenario and make healthy dessert sweet, use natural sweeteners like raw honey or maple syrup instead of refined sugar. You can also use ripe fruits; they tend to add a naturally sweet flavor to those healthy desserts.

Use high-quality ingredients

The quality of your dessert has a lot to do with the quality of the ingredients you have used. Therefore, make it your business to consider this and never compromise on quality. Are you now ready for healthy ice creams, cheesecakes, healthy pies, healthy frozen yogurts, and other awesome healthy desserts? You do not have to wait any longer, here are some of the best healthy desserts you can make for you and your family.

Chocolate chip gingerbread

These flourless ginger blondies made with high-protein chickpeas are vegan and gluten-free snack bars. They can make the perfect healthy treat for both kids and adults.

What you will need

- Drained chickpeas
- Almond butter/ Cashew butter
- Pure maple syrup
- Ground ginger
- Vanilla extract
- Blackstrap molasses
- Ground flaxseed
- Cloves

- Cinnamon
- Nutmeg
- Baking powder
- Salt
- Baking soda
- Chocolate chips

For the maple glaze
- Cashew butter
- Maple syrup
- Cinnamon
- Coconut oil
- Ground ginger

How to prepare

Preheat your oven to 350 Fahrenheit. Spray your cooking pan with coconut oil and cooking spray. In a large food processor, ass all the ingredients except the ones for glaze and process them until batter becomes very smooth. Two to three minutes should be enough, though. Then spread the batter evenly in the prepared pan. Evenly press the mixture into the pan using a spatula sprayed with cooking spray. Then bake the mixture for around twenty-five minutes.

Place the glaze ingredients in a small bowl and stir with a fork until they become very well combined. Ensure the coconut oil slightly melts as you stir. Set the mixture aside and allow the bars to cool. Then cut the cooled bars. Drizzle glaze onto bars.

Healthy no bake cherry vegan cheesecake

There is nothing complicated in making healthier desserts. One big secret is to substitute bad ingredients with healthy ingredients. The results are amazing. For instance, this healthy no bake cherry vegan cheesecake is made with a cashew-based filling, glutted-free crust and some delicious cherry layer on top. This is among the better tasting low-fat desserts that are as good as the classic ones.

Health benefits of cherries

Cherries and cheesecake offer a perfect combination. Further, cherries make a healthier no-bake cheesecake that you will love. Cherries are nutritious because they contain the following elements;

Melatonin

Studies indicate that cherries are filled with melatonin. The ingredient that helps your internal clock which regulates your normal sleep pattern.

Natural sweetness

The ideal dose of sweetness without unhealthy sugars is found in dark sweet or Rainier cherries. The reason as to why cherries are unique when compared with other fruits is that they contain a lower glycemic index in comparison to other fruits as they tend to release the glucose slowly and evenly.

As a result, this helps you to maintain a more stable blood sugar level, which leaves you feeling full for a longer time. This is also a plus to people who want to maintain a healthy weight.

Fiber

Cherries contain fiber, and they can assist you in reaching the recommended current dietary of two cups of fruit per day. More so, it can contribute to healthy weight maintenance, prevent diabetes and improve cardiovascular health. In addition to the above, cherries also contain vitamin A, vitamin C, calcium, antioxidants, iron, potassium and protein. Cherries are also fat-free, sodium-free, cholesterol-free and low in calories with just 87 calories in one cup. In general, consumption of cherries is healthy, and they are good for you. They can also make a perfect yummy treat and a tasty topping for a healthy cheesecake.

Best way to preserve cherries

In this particular case, the healthy no-bake cherry vegan cheesecake has been made using frozen cherries. Henceforth, you do not have to wait for the cherry season to make it. Make sure next time during fresh sweet cherries season you will go to the stores and grab as much as you will need before the next season. If you do so, you must have ways to preserve them without them losing their quality. This is very important since fresh cherries are rare to find during colder months. The best option is to preserve your cherries is to freeze them. However, before you consider buying frozen cherries in your local stores, be cautious since some are preserved with sugar and other unhealthy ingredients.

The only way to avoid this situation is to preserve them yourself. Do not worry, it is super easy to do so, and the results will excite you. You will also be able to control the ingredients used to preserve them. Nothing can be compared with taking control of what you feed yourself and your loved one with. On top of that, with all the outstanding cherry recipes, the meal can make all the year round if you decide to preserve the fresh sweet cherries, you have every reason to learn how to preserve them and enjoy all the benefits that come with it. Here are a couple of basic options you can use to preserve cherries:

Frozen cherries

The good thing about freezing cherries is that they freeze well. They can be used to make sweet smoothies and of course, cheesecake. To freeze them, you should place the frozen cherries on a baking dish on a single layer. Place them inside the freezer and then freeze until firm. You should then transfer all the contents inside a Ziploc bag. Once inside store them in the freezer; they will wait for you patiently until you need them.

Dry cherries

If you do not want to freeze your cherries, then you can opt to dry them. They also offer an amazing option to several recipes like baked cherry goods or granola. If you want to dry your cherries, you have options. You can always use a dehydrator or alternatively dry the cherries inside your oven.

Making the No-Bake Cherry Cheesecake

To make the no-bake cherry cheesecake, you will need to first get 3 ingredients, that is: crust, raw cashew filling and the sweet cherry topping with frozen cherries. Ideally, these are the basic steps one can use to in most cherry cheesecake recipes. However, in this case, things will be a bit different since this particular case involves making healthy cheesecake. The most impressive thing about this specific cheesecake, is you do not have to keep on worrying about the cooking duration for the cheesecake. Why? You will not have to do any cooking at all — no worries about oven heating issues and the like.

The ingredients required:

To pull out the crust you will need;

- Dates
- Raw pecans,
- Sea salt

To make the smooth, creamy filling you will need;

- Raw cashews,
- Lemon juice,
- Coconut oil,
- Pure maple syrup
- Coconut milk

The sweet cherry topping is made of;

- Frozen sweet cherries
- Water
- Lemon juice
- Pure maple syrup
- Arrowroot starch
- Lemon zest

Now that you know the ingredients, without further ado, let us learn how to make cherry cheesecake right away.

Begin by soaking the cashews inside boiling water for almost an hour. In the meantime, get your food processor, place the raw pecans, pitted dates and sea salt. Mix them until you create loose dough. Place it aside.

Next, take your loaf pan and then line it with parchment paper. Since this is a vegan no-bake cake, you will not be doing any baking. Just transfer your dough into a loaf pan.

Pack down the mixture using your fingers and there you have it. The cheesecake crust is now ready.

It is now time to check on the filling for the cheesecake. Drain all the soaked cashews. Then add them to the blender together with melted coconut oil, lemon juice, coconut milk, and maple syrup. Blend them until smooth. After that, pour your cheesecake filling on top of the cheesecake crust, then place it in the freezer.

You can now be working on the sweet cherry topping as your cheesecake settles in the freezer. To make it, simply begin by combining the cherries, water, lemon zest, lemon juice and the maple syrup inside a saucepan for around 12-15 minutes.

Then add the arrowroots starch and then whisk them together until the mixture turns smooth and then begins to thicken. Allow them to heat for another 2 minutes. Remove the mixture from the oven and then allow it to cool down to room temperature. Add it over the cheesecake. Feel free to taste what you just made!

Vegan matcha coconut tarts

Have you cooked with matcha before? If you have not yet, it is your high time you consider doing so. You should just roll up your sleeves and cook a tray of small matcha coconut tarts as soon as you can. This dessert is perfect for any season.

They are not only vegan but also gluten and refined sugar-free but better still; they are gorgeous and properly indulgent. They contain just the right amount of sweetness you need. If this is something you would love to give it a try, then why not, go ahead and make your matcha coconut tarts for your family.

What you will need:

Gluten-free pastry

Ingredients;

- Buckwheat flour
- Oats or oat flour
- Desiccated coconut
- Fine salt
- Tapioca starch or cornstarch
- Raw cacao powder
- Melted coconut oil
- Maple syrup

Matcha coconut filling

Ingredients;

- Soaked raw cashews
- Coconut cream
- Matcha powder
- Maple syrup
- Agar flakes or agar powder

How to make them

Use a coffee grinder or a food processor to grind oats and desiccated coconut into powder form.

Pre-heat the oven to 175/345 degrees F.

In a large bowl, put the ground coconut, buckwheat flour, oats, salt, tapioca, cacao, and starch. Stir them until they combine properly.

Add the melted coconut into the dry ingredients and rub it with your fingers. Add the maple syrup. Continue adding more oil and maple syrup until the mixture stops being too dry and comes together easily. Leave the dough for about 10 minutes.

Make sure you lubricate the ramekins with coconut oil. Once through with the greasing, you should then line the bottom of the pan with circles of baking paper. This will enable the tarts to come out easily after baking.

You should then divide the dough you just made into two equal portions and then press the dough into the sides and base of each ramekin. Ensure the dough is bound tightly together. Also, remember to press the dough gently to cover all the gaps.

After that, you can then bake it in the oven's middle shelf for about 16 minutes. Let the tarts cool down after baking and filling.

To make the filling, place the drained coconut cream, cashews, maple syrup and the matcha in a blender.

Then place the agar flakes inside a small pot, put some water and bring to a gentle boil. Simmer and then remember to stir frequently for around fifteen minutes or until the agar is almost dissolved.

Leave it to cool down a bit. There is no point of adding the agar to the remaining ingredients.

Add the warm agar mixture to your blender and then process the mixture until it becomes smooth. Give it about 3o minutes to set in. Your filling should be ready now.

Doughy peach pie bars

These doughy peach pie bars should be your favorite because apart from them being a healthy dessert, they are also suitable for breakfast or snacks. In other words, these bars are multipurpose. If peaches are not delicious to you, you can use bananas instead.

Ingredients needed

Bottom crust layer

- Oat Flour
- Salt
- Egg
- Greek yogurt
- Small cubes butter

Middle layer

- Thinly sliced peaches or bananas

Streusel topping

- Old-fashioned oats
- Finely chopped walnuts
- Melted butter
- Honey
- Cinnamon
- Salt

Directions to make

To make the bottom crust layer, combine salt, oat flour, honey, egg, and the Greek yogurt inside a bowl.

Add the cold butter to the ingredients in the bowl. Use your fingers to incorporate the butter into the dough. Although the dough with not get crumbly likes sand, it instead is the consistency of the biscuit dough.

Grease a casserole dish and press your dough inside. Then place the sliced peaches on the dough.

Now it is time to make the streusel topping. In a medium-sized bowl, combine the walnuts, oats, butter, cinnamon, honey, and salt. Sprinkle the streusel on the peaches — Bake the contents for about 18 minutes.

You can enjoy it warm or keep it in the fridge and eat it cold. In both situations, you will like it for sure.

No-bake blueberry custard pie (vegan and gluten-free)

This easy no-bake pie will brighten up your days when you are not in the mood to heat the oven, especially during summer days but still, want something fancy and yummy at the same time.

The beauty of vegan pie crusts is that they are super easy to make. They also contain healthy fat and tastes great too.

Plus, no baking is needed to enjoy this delicacy. As for the creamy vanilla custard filling, it is strictly vegan with almond milk.

Another interesting thing about this recipe is that you have the opportunity to make it a day or two ahead up to the crust/filling steps. Isn't it amazing? On the D-day, just throw the jam/blueberry mixture on top, and you are good.

You will not even believe its vegan and gluten-free when you finally taste it. All the growly goes to the crunchy crust, creamy vanilla filling and juicy blueberry topping. You just need to do your thing a few hours in advance, and everyone who tastes it will thank you a lot.

What you need for:

The crust:

- Raw walnuts
- Raw almonds
- Unsweetened shredded coconut
- Pitted dates

The filling:

- Vegan cane sugar
- Cornstarch
- Unsweetened vanilla
- Coconut oil
- Vanilla extract

The topping:

- Blueberry jam
- Fresh blueberries

Directions to make:

Process all the crust ingredients inside a food processor until they become finely ground. In a greased pan with a removable bottom, press the crust mixture inside. Set it aside.

Next, put sugar and cornstarch in a medium pot. Do so as you whisk to eliminate any lumps. Whisk the Almond Breeze inside the mixture.

Put the almond breeze mixture to medium to high heat and bring them to a gentle boil. Then adjust the heat from medium to low. Whilst the mixture vigorously until it thickens. This should take you about 3 to 5 minutes. Once the mixture is ready, remove the mixture from heat. Whisk in the coconut oil and vanilla extract.

Pour the filling onto the crust generously and gently, then leave it to cool. Once cool, use a plastic wrap to tightly wrap it and put it in the fridge for at least an hour, the longer, the better. If you don't intend on doing so much in just one day, you can always leave preparing the pie. It can always be consumed at this stage.

Next, melt the jam by warming it on the microwave. Spread all the liquid jam on the cooled filling. You can use a spatula or a spoon. Then top with fresh blueberries.

Banana chocolate and peanut butter swirl bread with pecan praline

Do you have overripe bananas in the house and are planning to throw them away? Please do not do that. Instead, consider giving this recipe a try, and you will love the outcome. The bread does taste so good that next time you will buy lots of bananas without the fear they will get spoilt.

What you will need:

- Gluten-free flour/All-purpose flour
- Baking powder
- Salt
- Baking soda
- Cinnamon
- Ripe bananas
- Creamy peanut butter
- Eggs
- Coconut oil
- Unsweetened applesauce
- Sugar
- Vanilla
- Semi-sweet chocolate chips

Pecan praline

- Brown sugar
- Butter
- Low-fat milk
- Chopped pecans
- Vanilla

How to make banana chocolate and peanut butter swirl bread

Preheat your oven to 370 degrees F. Use the cooking spray to spray the loaf pan and line it with parchment paper. The parchment paper makes the removing of the bread much easier.

Next, mix the baking powder, flour, baking soda, cinnamon, salt inside a medium-sized bowl.

In another bowl, mash the bananas until you see no chunks left. Then add in the sugar, eggs, oil, peanut butter, vanilla and applesauce. Gradually, mix gently the flour. Divide the butter into two bowls.

Put the chocolate chips inside the microwave to melt. The best way is to begin by heating it for around 30 seconds. Then continue heating the mixture at 15 seconds intervals. Do so, until all the chips turn glossy. You should then pull the chocolate chips from the microwave and immediately stir until you achieve a creamy-chocolate mixture.

Add the chocolate mixture to one half of the batter.

Take your loaf pan and pour the batter into it. Remember to alternate the dark and light batter. Swirl the batter on the top with the help of a knife, toothpick or a skewer. Simply create a pattern without overworking it.

Bake for about 55 to 60 minutes. You can test, using a toothpick. If it comes clean, then it's all ready. Allow the bread to cool for about 10 minutes. After that, you can remove it from the pan.

Then prepare the praline. Get a small saucepan and melt the butter. On the melted butter, add sugar and milk. Combine them thoroughly until you come up with something like a sauce. Remove from the heat and then stir in pecans and vanilla.

Now pour your sauce onto the bread. The praline tends to harden pretty faster.

In case it hardens before pouring it onto the bread, then you have to reheat it. However, this time around do it a bit faster. Any leftovers should be wrapped and refrigerated; they can last up to one week.

Dark chocolate almond oatmeal cookies with sea salt

Who said you must give up on your 3 pm cookie simply because you are **meal prep** for a healthier you? The truth is you do not have to, you just need to make a healthy recipe like this one, and all will be well.

These dark cookies are not something that you may want to overlook. They have got little extra protein and healthy fats thanks to the almond butter. They are also interesting and easy to make.

What you will need;

- Coconut oil
- Eggs
- Maple syrup
- Almond butter
- Rolled oats
- Vanilla
- Cinnamon
- Baking soda
- Dark chocolate
- Coarse sea salt

Instructions to make it

Begin by preheating the oven to about 350 degrees F. Line the baking pan with a parchment paper. Use a bowl to mix the coconut oil, eggs, maple syrup, vanilla and almond butter.

Using a large bowl, mix the cinnamon, rolled oats, dark chocolate, and baking soda. Mix the wet ingredients with the dry ones inside a large bowl. Stir them to combine. Make sure the dry mixture is evenly coated. Pour the dough into the baking sheet, leave some space between cookies. Then, sprinkle each with a few sea salt flakes. Bake the cake for around 12 minutes or alternatively until the cookies turn golden brown.

3-ingredient guilt free brownies

These brownies are gluten-free and vegan. Plus, they will take you not more than five minutes. No bake recipes are worth celebrating. Below are the 3 ingredients you will need;

- Dates pitted
- Cocoa powder
- Honey roasted vanilla
- water

If you like, you can add additional flavors such as vanilla, sea salt, chocolate chips, shredded coconut, seeds and the like.

How to make it:

Begin by placing the almonds in the food processor and coarsely chop. Remove and set aside.

Next, put the dates in the same food processor and coarsely chop. Add water and cocoa powder and process until combined like cookie dough. Add the almond and whisk until relatively combined. Transfer the mixture into a bowl and finish combining by kneading the dough into a bowl.

Get a piece of parchment on your counter top and roll dough into a 1/3 of an inch thick slab. Then cut them into square or your desired shape.

If you intend to keep them for longer, you can keep yours in a Tupperware in the freezer. You can do so by putting them on a baking sheet with a piece of parchment paper and freeze them. Then transfer them into the Tupperware. This way, they can last longer, and they taste sweeter when frozen. However, do not be restricted by this; you can also do it your way.

Creamy lime and avocado tart

You should try adding these tarts to your meal prep rotation. They are so tasty but healthy at the same time. After having a bite, you will wonder what you have been doing all this while without cooking these awesome creamy lime and avocado tart. If you have opted to make a mini cupcake, make sure that the tarts are frozen when getting them out of the cupcake tin least you ruin them up.

The tarts are best served when frozen. After removing them in the freezer, you can allow them to thaw for around 10 minutes before serving. If you like the frozen texture, then go ahead and try them before the 10 minutes. You should test to see which form works best for your taste buds. However, if you leave the tarts unfrozen for some time, the filling will eventually get extremely soft, much similar to pudding. Henceforth, make sure you freeze any leftovers. The beauty of these tarts is that they are made using natural ingredients. They are also full of healthy fats from avocados, pecans and coconut. They are vegan, gluten-free and creamy. Do you want to try them? Below are the ingredients you will need and how to make them.

What you will need:

Crust:

- Shredded unsweetened coconut
- Chopped pecans
- Dates
- Lime zest

Tart filling

- Avocados
- Freshly squeezed lime juice
- Coconut or honey
- Coconut oil
- Lime zest

How to make it:

Use a food processor to process the ingredients including pecans, coconut, lime zest, dates and sea salt. You can also use a mini chopper. The point is to ensure the dates have converted into a sticky paste so that they can hold the crust ingredients. Remove the mixture from the processor and evenly press it inside two mini springform pans. Place the pans in the freezer. In the meantime, you can be making the tart filling. Blend the avocados, lime juice, agave, coconut oil and lime zest. Do so in a high-speed blender or better still a food processor until the mixture becomes creamy.

Pour the avocado filling over the crust in the two pans. Use a spoon or a spatula to evenly spread the mixture. Place the pans in the freezer for not less than 2 hours, overnight is best. Take it out of the freezer, remove the pan and allow it to sit for 10 to 15 minutes. Then cut into the desired size and serve. Remember to store any leftovers in the freezer.

Vegan brown rice crispy treats

Healthy brown rice treats are not only vegan but also gluten-free. They are made using brown rice syrup, almond butter and coconut oil. Instead of feeding your loved ones with marshmallow based rice crispy treats, why don't you replace that with a healthier option? To add a little bit of fun, you can always add a few dairy-free chocolate chips. However, if you prefer a lower amount of sugar, it is better you forego the chocolate chips. The brown rice cereal is gluten-free since it's made using whole grain brown rice. You can find it in most health food stores. The brown rice syrup is a natural sweetener that has a much low glycemic index. It is also available in your local healthy food store. Although you can use maple syrup, in this particular recipe, brown rice syrup tends to perform better. Its thick and sticky nature helps it to hold the treats together nicely. These treats are great for desserts or snacks. They can be enjoyed by both adults and kids. Without further ado, here is the recipe.

What you will need:

- Brown rice syrup
- Coconut oil
- Almond butter
- Vanilla extract
- Brown rice crisp cereal
- Sea salt
- Dairy-free mini chocolate chips (optional)

How to make it:

Place the brown rice crisp cereal onto a bowl.

Next, place brown almond butter, rice syrup and the coconut oil in a saucepan on medium heat. Heat and stir until the mixture is well combined and creamy. 5 minutes should be okay. Once ready, remove the mixture from heat and then add vanilla and a little bit sea salt. Pour the mixture onto the rice cereal and then stir until everything is well combined. Line your baking dish using a parchment paper. Press the chocolate chips onto the top. Put it in the fridge for about an hour. Remove and cut into desired shapes.

Chapter 4: Snack meal prepping

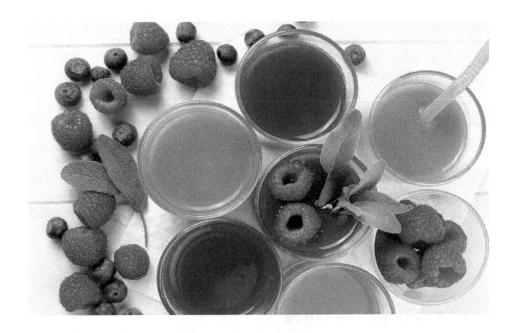

Snacks are those little meals you indulge in throughout the day between breakfast, lunch, and dinner. Snacking is a good thing, and it can help you to re-energize when you feel worn out. You need healthy and nutritious little snacks here and there throughout the day.

Snacks are sometimes forbidden for being sugary, salty and empty calories. However, snacks do not have to be unhealthy. For instance, carrots and hummus are popular snacks since they provide protein and easily fill a part of your veggie quota for the day.

Below are benefited your body gets to enjoy when you make it a habit to snack throughout the day. Therefore, go ahead and grab a snack and do not feel guilty about it.

1. Provides diverse nutrients

Apart from eating three square meals a day, snacking in between meals is a very healthy lifestyle choice. Snacking can help increase your nutrient intake and allow you to get many benefits from the different types of food you are taking. Adding healthy snacks to your regular meals can help your body to benefit from nutrients such as vitamins, proteins and fiber.

2. Prevents binge eating

One big mistake people do is an attempt to deny them something to snack for so long that when they eventually decide to eat, they end up reaching for something unhealthy. There is nothing wrong with snacking, and so you do not have to feel guilty when you.

When you deny yourself something to snack for a longer time, most probably you end up having unhealthy cravings. More so, it makes sustaining a healthy lifestyle seem like an unachievable task. Hence, it is better to snack on filling foods in between meals. It will keep you satisfied throughout the day.

3. Beats the afternoon slump

The late-afternoon slump is a difficult thing to defeat for sure. Fighting your fatigue until dinner time can be a nightmare as it leads to sluggishness and low productivity.

Fortunately, this is something you can avoid by treating yourself to something with something to eat in between meals. It will take your energy to the required level.

4. Raises metabolism

When your body is constantly busy processing food, turns into a well-oiled machine. Snacking on healthy snacks will also keep your ticker and bloodstream pumping away. This greatly improves your body from inside. So, next time you are told to eat fewer meals to keep fit, do not forget that your metabolism requires energy to function regularly and be the best it needs to be.

5. Increases concentration

When you snack on healthy snacks in between meals, your level of concentration also increases. As a result, learning in school or getting work done in the office becomes easier. Eating snacks helps you to feel full, sharp and alert throughout the day.

Healthy meal prep snacks

Although some planning and preparation are required to stay on the path of healthy snacking, the benefits are worth it. Meal prep is not about lunch and dinner only; it also involves snacks. If you find it hard to eat well during the day as you run errands, stay on track by knowing how to meal healthy prep snacks. The possibilities snack meal prepping are almost endless. Here are just a few ideas to help you get started.

1. **Bananas and peanut butter**

This combination is just amazing. They are a little sweet, a little salty and have a whole lot of potassium and protein. Do not underestimate them because of their small size. They have what it takes to give you a huge burst of energy to keep going throughout the day. To prepare them, remove the banana cover, cut it into medium sizes. Then apply peanut butter on one side of the banana and combine two pieces. If peanut butter and bananas are not your favorites, you can replace bananas with apples. This snack is equal parts crunchy and smooth.

If you want more crunches, then consider putting apple slices and a smear of peanut butter on crisp bread. You can pack them to work or school.

2. Avocado hummus snack jars

There is nothing super convenient like having something nutritious and delicious you can easily grab out of the fridge. It helps you keep on track with your health and wellness goals even when time is not on your side. This is a healthy snack idea that can serve such a purpose.

What you will need to prepare it

- Rinsed and drained chickpeas
- Tahini
- Diced avocado
- Minced garlic
- Lemon juice
- Salt
- Water
- Sliced sundried tomatoes (optional)
- Carrot sticks
- Celery sticks
- Cucumber
- Assorted cracks

How to prepare it

Add all the ingredients except veggies, avocado, and crackers to your blender. Blend them on the lowest speed in intervals of about 30 seconds. Remove the lid and stir. Continue with the process until fully mixed. The whole process should take you about 5 minutes.

Pour into jam jars and top with avocado or sundried tomatoes. You can serve alongside cut up veggies, crackers, chips or any healthy snack you have been craving for.

3. Popcorn

There are so many benefits associated with making popcorn become your number one snack option. First of all, they are easy to munch on, light and whole grain can be extremely healthy. Not all popcorns are healthy, though. To know exactly what you are consuming, it is better you air-pop your own so that you can know exactly what is in it. Further, homemade popcorn is quick and easy to make. Make some on Sunday and have something to snack on the whole week ahead.

4. Vanilla cashew butter cups

This delicious easy to make vanilla cashew butter cups can serve as healthy desserts and snacks.

Ingredients needed:

- Dark chocolate chips
- Cashew butter
- Honey or maple syrup
- Vanilla sea salt
- Flaky sea salt for the tops

How to prepare

Begin by lining the mini muffin tin with liners

Place 2/3 of the chocolate in a pan over low heat. Then remove it immediately it becomes glossy and melted. Add the remaining chocolate and stir a few times as the residual heats the just added chocolate.

Add some of the melted chocolate to one of the cupcake liners. Make sure the chocolate comes goes up the side of the liner by tipping it on its side and rotating it.

Repeat the same to all the liners. Place them in your fridge to harden.

Add the honey/maple syrup, cashew butter, vanilla, and salt to a bowl and gently combine them.

Once the chocolate cups have hardened, divide the cashew butter between the cups. Press it into the cup with your fingers or a spatula.

You can pour the remaining chocolate over the tops of the cashew butter cups and put them into your fridge until they harden. Finally, sprinkle a little flaky sea salt on top to make them irresistible.

Important things to note

If you have a microwave, you can use it to melt the chocolate. 20 to 30 seconds should be enough.

If you follow a vegan diet, make sure you read the label on the chocolate to see if it is okay for you to eat it.

Cashew nuts can be pricey. Save your cash by making your own using a food processor or a high powered blender.

Chapter 5: Vegan meal prep high protein

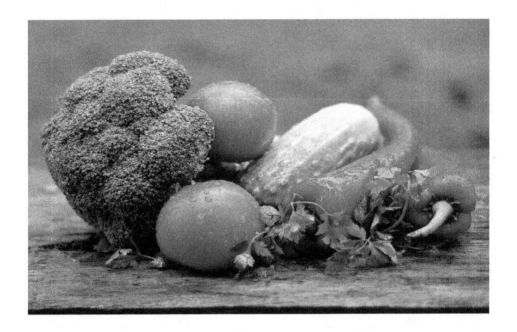

Are you wondering where vegans get their protein? Well, you are not alone. Most people ask this question a lot. What they do not know is that there are tons of protein sources in a vegan diet. Getting the amount you need is also easy. Plus, you do not have to achieve it by eating copious amounts of beans.

Below are a mixture of breakfasts, lunches, dinners, desserts and snacks recipes. They are most suitable to all those who are looking for proteins, healthy and gluten-free diet options.

Easy vegan chili sin carne

This is very easy to make delicacy as it will take you less than an hour to cook it. Further, if you are running out of time and want to make it extra easy, you can buy ready-prepared soffrito mixes at the food stores in the fresh veg or frozen section. This recipe involves a mixture of pre-chopped onion, celery and carrots. It is a very handy mixture to have in your fridge for soups, veggie Bolognese and the like. It is also packed with plant-based protein. You can make it in big portions for later servings. Here is the recipe.

What you will need:

- Olive oil
- Minced garlic
- Thinly sliced red onion
- Finely chopped celery stalks
- Peeled and finely chopped carrots
- Roughly chopped red pepper
- Ground cumin
- Chili powder
- Salt and pepper
- Tinned chopped tomatoes
- Red kidney beans
- Split red lentils
- Frozen soy mince
- Vegetables

How to make it:

Begin by heating the oil inside a saucepan.

Using medium heat, onion, sauté the garlic, celery, carrots and pepper for a few minutes. Then add cumin, chili powder, salt and pepper. Stir the mixture.

Pour in the chopped tomatoes, kidney beans, lentils, soy mince and vegetable stock. If you want to use any extra flavoring, this is the time to add it.

Simmer for 25 minutes. You can then serve it with rice, some freshly torn coriander and a squeeze of lime juice. You can also keep it in the fridge for up to 4 days.

High protein salad

This salad is the answer you seek if you have been looking for high protein, healthy salads recipes. The question of how vegans get protein is well answered. It is a great recipe for home snacks. You can also take with you to work, college or school.

What you will need:

For the salad;

- Canned green kidney beans (you use red ones as well)
- Canned lentils
- Arugula
- Capers

For the dressing

- Caper brine
- Tahini
- Peanut butter
- Tamari
- Hot sauce
- Balsamic vinegar

How to prepare it:

Add all the ingredients inside a bowl and whisk together until they combine to form a smooth dressing.

To make the salad, mix beans, lentils, arugula and capers. Top the meal with dressing and then enjoy your healthy meal.

Mexican lentil soup

The Mexican lentil soup is a tasty, nourishing, vegetarian and heart-healthy meal. It is indeed a complete one-pot meal. Both green and red lentils are a great protein source. You can then top the soup with several ingredients to add lots of flavors. Try it and who knows, it could be your new way to enjoy lentils.

What you will need:

- Extra virgin olive oil
- Diced yellow onion
- Peeled carrots
- Celery diced
- Diced red bell pepper
- Minced garlic
- Cumin
- Smoked paprika
- Oregano
- Diced tomatoes
- Diced green chilies
- Green lentils
- Vegetable Broth
- Salt
- Hot sauce
- Fresh cilantro, for garnish
- Avocado, peeled, pitted and diced

How to make it:

Inside a large pot, heat olive oil on medium heat. Then add carrots, onions, bell pepper and celery. Sauté for about 5 minutes or until they soften. Add cumin, garlic, oregano and paprika. Sauté for a minute.

Add tomatoes, chilies, lentils, broth and salt. Bring to simmer until lentils become tender. 30 to 40 minutes should be enough — season with pepper.

You can serve your lentil soup topped with avocado, fresh cilantro and dashes of hot sauce.

Black bean and quinoa balls

The quinoa balls are rich in flavor and delicious. Plus, you just need a few ingredients, and they are super easy to make. They go well with pasta or spiralized zucchini. You can also have them as snacks with your favorite dip.

This recipe is easy, quick, oil-free and healthy.

What you will need:

For the quinoa and the black bean;
- Quinoa
- Sesame seeds
- Black beans
- Oat Flour
- Sriracha
- Tomato paste
- Nutritional yeast
- Chopped fresh herbs
- Garlic powder
- Pepper
- Salt

For the sun-dried tomato sauce

- Sun-dried tomatoes
- Halved cherry tomatoes
- Garlic
- Apple cider vinegar
- Nutritional yeast
- Toasted pine nuts
- Oregano
- Fresh basil
- Pepper
- Salt

How to make it:

Add quinoa and water in a pot. Cook them for 15 minutes. You then drain any excess water and allow it to cool down for sometimes.

In the meantime, add a handful of black beans to the bowl and then mash them coarsely. Use a fork or a masher. Add sesame seeds, quinoa, oat flour, Sriracha, tomato paste, spice and nutritional yeast. Mix them well together. Make it into moldable dough.

Then roll the dough into small, tiny balls. Place the tiny balls on a baking sheet that is lined with baking paper — Bake for 35 to 40 minutes or until crispy.

Prepare your pasta the way you like it or according to the directions on the package.

For the tomato sauce, place the ingredients inside a food processor and then blend the ingredients until they turn creamy.

To serve, pasta with a few balls on each serving and then sprinkle them with fresh basil.

Chapter 6: Vegan meal prep weight loss

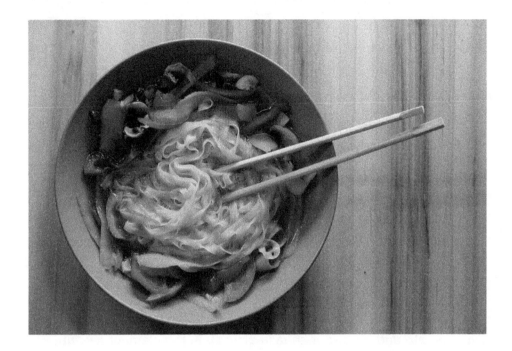

To maintain optimal health as a vegan is achievable.

Begin by ensuring you select fresh, seasonal unprocessed, locally sourced organic foods.

Here are the key ingredients that you will need to include to your healthy vegan plan;

1. Whole grains

Oats and brown rice are a great source of iron, and they can also keep you satisfied for longer as compared to the processed options. Foods made in grains are full of fiber. Hence, consider increasing your intake of millet, amaranth, barley and faro. They will keep you full and reduce your intake of unhealthy snacking.

2. Vegetables

Vegetables such as collard greens, kale and spinach are widely known to boost one's iron levels. Further, you squeeze some fresh lemon juice; your body will receive enough vitamin C to accelerate your iron absorption.

Sweet potato and butternut squash are rich in the element calcium and with them, you can forget about consuming dairy products. As for broccoli, cauliflower and Brussels sprouts, they are part of cruciferous family best known as cancer superheroes.

3. Legumes (soy, beans, and lentils)

Legumes form the base of a vegan meal plan. Legumes will deliver more than enough plant-based protein to your body, and this keeps your metabolism running.

You also get strong muscles and most importantly, you do not feel the urge to grab any processed treats since you will not feel hungry.

Soy products such as soy milk or tofu tempeh are foods that greatly supports your weight loss efforts. However, they give the best results when consumed in their unprocessed and unsweetened state.

4. Healthy Fats

Who said you enjoy intake of fats if you are losing weight. So long as they are healthy fats, you do not have to feel guilty indulging your favorite dish or snack. For instance, avocado and olive oil contain high levels of vitamin E, which is beneficial to healthy skin. Besides, they also have high levels of monounsaturated fats. Walnuts and Ground flaxseeds are high in omega-3 fats, an anti-inflammatory whose task is to assist the body release excess water or toxins.

5. Nuts, nut butter, and milk

If you want healthy snacks to grab as you head out, then go for walnuts, peanuts, almonds, cashews, pistachios and hazelnuts. They are not only super tasty, but they are also high in protein and calcium. When you consume them, you fill full for a longer time and so you will not eat too much.

6. Berries, apples, and bananas

Berries are very beneficial to your body. They protect you from inflammation and cancer. Moreover, they assist your skin to stay young-looking and supple. As for bananas, they form a great component for a vegan meal plan either for sweetening or baking.

Although bananas are high in soluble fiber, control your intake as they are still high in sugar. Apples are also essential to your weight loss journey as they contain pectin, a substance which tends to feed on the healthy bacteria found inside the gut. A healthy gut often translates to a much healthy weight.

Tips to lose weight as a vegan

According to research, individuals who follow a vegan diet can loose weight having a higher chance in comparison to those who are animal-based diets user. If you also want to loose some weight, below are tips that can help you do just that.

1. Eat greens

An addition of greens such as broccoli, spinach, chard, swiss, bok choy, zucchini and Brussels sprouts to your meal is crucial. Their greens are ideal for weight loss since they are extremely low in calories and high in fiber.

The high-content in fiber makes sure you feel full for a longer time, and this helps you to avoid unhealthy snacking. Other high-fiber options you can consider are fruits and raw tree nuts such as walnuts, almonds and cashews. They can also help lower cholesterol.

2. Increase your protein intake

If you intend to lose some extra pounds, then up your protein intake. Foods rich in protein helps you to feel full up faster. Thus, with just a little food, you will feel satisfied. Because proteins are readily available in different forms, it is convenient to incorporate them into your meals since you can have them in their row forms or cooked. For breakfasts and mid-day smoothie, you can have protein powders. The other plant-based proteins like beans, tempeh lentils oats and quinoa can be used to serve the main elements of a burrito, veggie, stir-fry or salad.

3. Limit processed soy

When a transition to a vegan diet, soy products comes in handy as they are the easiest and most convenient items you can grab on your way. This does not mean soy is unhealthy, not at all. However, it is important you limit the processed soy. For instance, instead of a tofu scramble for breakfast, soy veggies burger for lunch and a pad Thai with tofu for dinner, why can't go for vegan cheese made with nuts, a black bean burger or even a pad Thai with veggies?

4. Prepare healthy meals

Meal planning has a lot to do when it comes to proper nutrition and weight loss. If time is not on your side, you can prepare easy dishes such as quinoa bowls; a mixed stir-fry blend of carrots, broccoli and mushrooms, vegan cheese, eggplant cutlets with a little bit of marinara sauce and soba noodles. Plus do not be limited to this; you can also get more easy-to-follow recipes that are dietitian approved.

5. Stay hydrated and exercise.

The key components of a successful weight loss program must incorporate healthy meals, water and exercise. To burn calories and lose weight, you should engage in 150 minutes of moderate aerobic activity or 75 minutes of vigorous aerobic activity in a week.

Conclusion

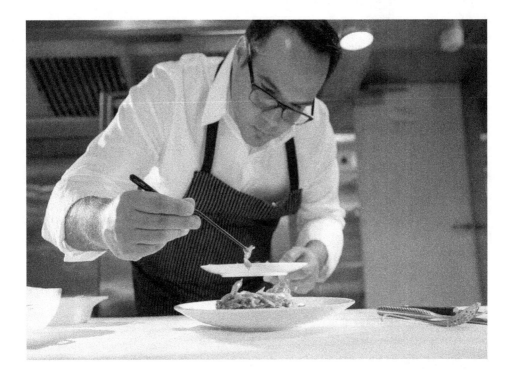

Thank you for making it through to the end of **_Vegan Meal Prep_**, let's hope it was informative and able to provide you with all of the tools you need to achieve your goals whatever they may be.

The next step is to highlight the best parts of the book that you would not want to miss.

Here's what you learned:

- Knowing what exactly is vegan meal prepping
- Best tips for meal prepping
- Safe and healthy tips for storing your food
- Vegan meal prepping for breakfast
- Vegan meal prepping for lunch and dinner
- Vegan meal prep for weight loss
- Things to consider when choosing a recipe
- Dessert meal prepping
- Snack meal prepping
- How to save time while meal prepping
- Best ways to feed yourself and loved ones with healthy meals the whole week

This book will greatly help you to make maximum use of the free time you have on weekends to prepare healthy and delicious meals that will be eaten throughout the week. The book is meant to help you cope with tight schedules like a pro. Life becomes much easier and interesting when meals are ready and what is required of you is just a few minutes to serve dinner or breakfast.

Plus, you can also have readily available snacks to grab on the go. All these things are possible, and you can make life much enjoyable if you take your time to go through this Book.

In general, when you read this book and learn different *vegan meal prep* recipes, the results will be impressive. The ideas will help you save time. After a day of *meal prep*, things will be much easier the following days. There will be fewer dishes and plates to clean and less time to spend in the kitchen as dinner can be ready in minutes.

It will also help you create healthy eating habits for you and your family. Healthy eating is about being prepared, and if you have readily prepared meals for the week, nothing will stop you from eating healthy.

It will also be easier for you to eat a balanced diet and this is very beneficial to your overall health. This book will also help you reduce stress. When you know that your family has something to eat for dinner, you will be able to relax and concentrate more on what you are doing.

Finally, if you found this book useful in any way, a five star review is always appreciated !

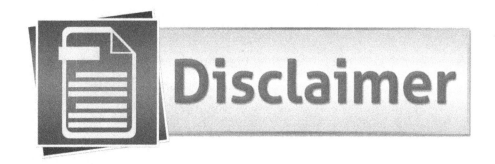